Traditional
Chinese Medicine

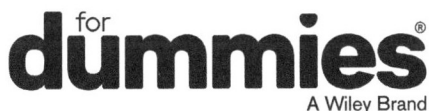

A Wiley Brand

Traditional
Chinese Medicine

by Dr. Mi-Yung L. Rhee, DACM,
Dipl. O.M. (NCCAOM)®, L.Ac.

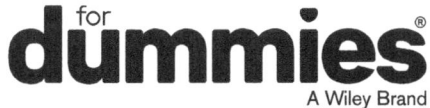

Traditional Chinese Medicine For Dummies®

Published by: **John Wiley & Sons, Inc.,** 111 River Street, Hoboken, NJ 07030-5774, www.wiley.com

For general information on our other products and services, please contact our Customer Care Department within the U.S. at 877-762-2974, outside the U.S. at 317-572-3993, or fax 317-572-4002. For technical support, please visit https://hub.wiley.com/community/support/dummies.

Wiley publishes in a variety of print and electronic formats and by print-on-demand. Some material included with standard print versions of this book may not be included in e-books or in print-on-demand. If this book refers to media that is not included in the version you purchased, you may download this material at http://booksupport.wiley.com. For more information about Wiley products, visit www.wiley.com.

Library of Congress Control Number is available from the publisher.

ISBN 978-1-394-28459-7 (pbk); ISBN 978-1-394-28462-7 (ebk); ISBN 978-1-394-28460-3 (ebk)

Printed and bound by CPI Group (UK) Ltd, Croydon CR0 4YY

C9781394284597_040326

The manufacturer's authorized representative according to the EU General Product Safety Regulation is Wiley-VCH GmbH, Boschstr. 12, 69469 Weinheim, Germany, e-mail: Product_Safety@wiley.com.

Contents at a Glance

Table of Contents

Introduction

When I resigned from my lucrative marketing position to return to school in 2010, I fully expected someone in my trusted circle of family, friends, and mentors to tell me, "You're crazy!" When I told them I was going to study Traditional Chinese Medicine, I fully expected to hear, "You've lost your mind."

> FLASHBACK: I lost my mind in 2006 after my father's triple bypass surgery. I was at my parents' kitchen table sorting his medication into weekly pill organizers. Gazing at the different hues of pink, blue, yellow, and cream, I realized he would take and process over 200,000 of these pills in his remaining lifetime.
>
> I was a little dismayed that no one questioned or tried to point out the lack of logic in this plan — only treating his medical issues with prescriptions. You see, I was ready to dive into researching other options at the first word of caution or a Mr. Spock-like brow tilt from my family.
>
> I thought, "There's got to be more than this." It took three years of research for me to find the solution and another year to implement it.

If you're holding this book in your hands or perusing its pages on a tablet, you know my plan of seeking knowledge came to fruition. I traded my six-figure job for a five-figure student loan and two post-graduate degrees.

I wrote this book from my perspective when I first set foot in a classroom at the American College of Traditional Medicine in San Francisco. Although I wish I could say I never looked back or had any doubts (there were plenty), I haven't regretted taking the leap.

About This Book

As a Traditional Chinese Medicine (TCM) practitioner, you follow a path of channels in the body that are associated with the Five Elements and theories such as Yin and Yang, which I discuss in Chapter 2. Then you get a whiff of a decocted herbal brew and officially enter a kind of wonderland — where the careful insertion of a hair-thin acupuncture needle in the crook of an elbow can help to reduce fever and calm a cough.

For the uninitiated, which I assume is why you're here, you may find this result hard to believe. So, *Traditional Chinese Medicine For Dummies* will take you on a not-so-magical, but still mysterious tour of Traditional Chinese Medicine.

Although you can certainly find other books (and the Internet) to provide you with information about TCM, most of those sources are textbooks for students, deep dives into one aspect of TCM theory or technique, or applications of TCM to a specific condition. Some are missing information that a potential patient might want or need.

In this book, I provide you with enough information to make a reasoned decision about supporting your health with TCM, in addition to historical perspectives and theories. Organized in an easy-to-access format, the book is divided into four parts:

>> Part 1 is aptly an overview of TCM as a healing system with its origins, techniques, theories, and practitioner licensing.

>> Part 2 provides more details about TCM treatments and therapies.

>> Part 3 discusses the application of TCM to a range of common health issues or conditions — from physical pain to mental health.

>> Part 4 gives you some opportunities to take baby steps to integrate some TCM into your self-care routine.

The table of contents is your road map on this mystery tour, and you can pretty much start anywhere you like. But I recommend that you start with TCM theory and practitioner credentials in Part 1 because this is like learning to read, write, and speak a new language. Part 1 represents the alphabet — the individual components that come together in various combinations to form different words. The TCM therapies and treatments in Part 2 are the words that are determined by the alphabet. Finally, in Part 3, the words become sentences as TCM therapies are used for specific ailments and illnesses. If you pick up new languages easily, you can skip the words in Part 2. Frankly, I'm a word geek, so I think the best part of learning a new language is mastering the vocabulary to produce the best sentences.

I've tried to minimize jargon and unfamiliar words throughout the book. However, TCM and medicine overall have their own terminology, so you can expect some unfamiliar words when you're just starting out. Within the text, I define terms briefly, and the Glossary (see Appendix A) provides all the terms (and TCM-related organizations) in one spot at the end of the book. The resources in Appendix B include sites where you can find more detailed information about health conditions discussed in the chapters.

Throughout this book, I've capitalized TCM terms for the organs (Kidney, Lung, Spleen, and others). When these terms appear in lowercase (kidney, lung, spleen, and others), I'm using Western medical terminology.

Foolish Assumptions

I'm guessing you've picked up this book because you're curious about Traditional Chinese Medicine.

Perhaps you've heard about acupuncture, but you have a fear of needles. Or maybe you had a negative experience with acupuncture and are considering giving it another shot — no pun intended! Maybe you or someone you care about is facing some health challenges, and a fistful of pills doesn't appeal to you. Or whatever you're doing for your own health isn't working, and you're ready to explore other options.

Whatever your reasons are for reading this book, I've made a couple of other foolish assumptions that may reflect your viewpoint:

>> You're open to new health-care approaches and are ready to take steps to control your health destiny.

>> You're unsure about TCM, but you're arming yourself with information that you can use to advocate for yourself to ask questions of your providers so that they can serve you better.

Icons Used in This Book

Throughout this book, icons in the margins highlight certain types of valuable information that deserve your attention. Here are the icons that you'll encounter and a brief description of each.

This icon indicates where I express a personal opinion or share my perspective on a topic from my own experience.

The Tip icon marks actions you can take to better prepare for a TCM treatment and other general health information.

REMEMBER

Remember icons highlight information that's important to know so that you can skim the text for the really meaty bits if you want.

TECHNICAL
STUFF

The Technical Stuff icon marks information that may be interesting to know, but you won't lose out if you skip it.

WARNING

The Warning icon signals important information that relates to safety, legal, or troublesome issues. You don't have to read every word in this book, but don't miss these paragraphs.

The sidebars that appear in the book include information that is related to or expands upon the subject at hand. Like Technical Stuff, you won't miss anything critical if you skip them. However, there's one at the beginning of Chapter 13 that you should read.

Beyond the Book

In addition to the abundance of information and guidance related to Traditional Chinese Medicine that I provide in this book, you get access to even more help and information online at Dummies.com. Check out this book's online Cheat Sheet. Just go to www.dummies.com and search for "Traditional Chinese Medicine For Dummies Cheat Sheet."

Where to Go from Here

If this book piques your interest in learning more about TCM or any of its components, you might start as I did. I took a four-class introduction to TCM at one of the local Bay Area colleges that was designed for the general public. Of course, this was pre-COVID, so I don't know what's available now. I'd recommend looking for a local school and contacting them to ask if they offer classes for the general public. Finally, the best way to learn more about TCM is to see a practitioner and experience it for yourself. Thank you for letting me share my journey with you.

1
Getting Started with TCM

Discover how Traditional Chinese Medicine (TCM) compares with Western medicine as a healing system in its origins and therapies

Gain an understanding of the basic theories and concepts behind TCM's approach to illness, anatomy, and healing

Find out how credentials and licensing maintain the competency of practitioners and the safety of patients so that you can choose a practitioner who best fits your needs

Chapter **1**

Looking at Health through a TCM Lens

When I was growing up, I tried to fake a fever by putting my forehead under the desk lamp to get out of school. But I was rarely successful because my father was a doctor. He'd place his hand on my forehead, look down my throat, and pronounce me fit to go. He was the one who calmly explained why I wasn't dying when I woke with blood between my legs in the middle of the night at age 12. Neighbors and church members sought him out for medical advice, and he was spot on with his diagnosis. I thought he always wanted to be a doctor. It wasn't until I was an adult that I learned his choice of profession was born from personal tragedy during the Korean War.

His older brother, a college freshman, bled to death from shrapnel wounds when a bomb hit outside the front gate of their family home. My father, a high school senior, watched him die in his mother's arms and helped bury him in the backyard. This is why my father became a doctor instead of an architect or filmmaker as his heart desired.

My father's heart surgery and later onset of Parkinson's disease prompted my own exploration of an alternative to his colorful parade of pills (see the Introduction). I was also restless in my career and questioned if I wanted to retire on deadlines in front of a computer.

I share this because not every fork in the road is a choice. Sometimes, the path you take is more necessity than destiny. I never imagined following in my father's footsteps because math and science were a slog for me. (Confession: I got through biology without ever dissecting anything. I had my lab partner do it.) Necessity presented itself with my father's health and my personal career conundrum. And I steered as far from medicine as I could until I discovered the medicine I'd like to introduce to you in this book.

Stepping out of my comfort zone was simultaneously exciting and scary. But whenever I've reached a crossroads in my life — big or small — I've turned to my favorite poem, *The Road Not Taken*, by Robert Frost. My interpretation of it has been my guiding philosophy as an adult.

However, when it comes to any kind of health care, I like to move forward with an annotated map that contains as much information about the routes that I have available to reach my destination. For example, when I was diagnosed with osteo-arthritis (wear-and-tear cartilage loss) in my right hip, my doctor and I discussed the options available to me to manage my pain and improve my range of motion, including steroid shots, pain medication, physical therapy, and strength training, with surgery as the last stop on the treatment train. I declined the steroid shots and pain medication and went to physical therapy, strength training, and yoga. With my doctor's agreement, I also incorporated acupuncture, tui na, and Traditional Chinese Herbs (TCH). (See Chapters 4 and 5.) As a result, I went 11 months before reaching my last stop of hip replacement surgery. To top it off, my recovery was minimally painful (2 out of 10 on the pain scale without any opioid medication) and faster than anticipated (fully mobile with a cane in three weeks).

So, if your health-care approach aligns with mine, I hope this book can serve as part of your map and offer you some options that you may not have considered before.

Recognizing TCM as a System of Healing

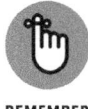

REMEMBER

The phrase *Traditional Chinese Medicine* (TCM) is a misnomer. Perhaps *East Asian Medicine* or *Asian-Inspired Medicine* are more accurate terms because, as practiced in the Western world, TCM also incorporates techniques, styles, and approaches from other Asian countries, Europe, and the U.S. — not just China. The term TCM is widely used around the world (in media, research, education, and medical and health-related institutions), so that's the term I use.

TCM is based on a theoretical framework that seeks to explain how the human body functions, behaves, and reacts within the expansive ecosystem of life on this planet. The framework is built on theories and concepts about the human condition and health that guide where, when, why, and how practitioners should apply TCM techniques. I give you a sliver of insight into this framework in Chapter 2.

Western medicine (also known as allopathic medicine, biomedicine, or conventional medicine) is predominately used by doctors in private practice and hospitals within the United States. It's also the global standard. Its roots lie in Greece, which is considered Western (even though it's both east and west of the North American continent, depending on which way the crow flies). As described by the Cleveland Clinic, "This type of medical care uses techniques based on scientific evidence."

To distinguish TCM from Western medicine, you can categorize TCM's treatments and approaches in three ways. TCM involves healing:

» Naturally

» Holistically

» Integratively

I discuss each category briefly in the following sections.

Healing naturally

The most common definitions for *natural* relate to something existing in nature or caused by nature — more specifically, not made or caused by humans. (I find this concept difficult to reconcile because humans *are* natural beings, but I digress.)

If you search online for "natural healing," your results offer information about acupuncture, tai chi, and herbal remedies, along with other nonsurgical, non-pharmaceutical treatment methods such as meditation, massage, homeopathy, naturopathy, and aromatherapy. What many health-related websites don't acknowledge often (or at all) is that acupuncture, tai chi, herbal prescriptions, and so on are part of an entire system of TCM medicine.

At this time in human history, I think TCM's prime directive is to remind the body to do what its form, adaptations, and evolution allow it to do — to protect and heal itself naturally.

Healing holistically

TCM falls into the category labeled *holistic medicine,* which is based on the novel idea that a person's health involves not just their physical wellness, but also their mental, emotional, and spiritual wellness. Some osteopaths, chiropractors, and naturopaths call it a *whole-body approach.* (Although I can't imagine what a *partial-body approach* even looks like.)

Widely acknowledged as the father of medicine, Hippocrates established many of the standards of clinical medicine today. Hippocratic doctors consider each person to be unique. As part of their consult, they consider a patient's age, gender, appearance, physique, daily habits, where they live, and even the season of the year. This focus on the individual characteristics of a patient differs from Western medicine's focus on the patient's symptoms.

Hippocrates' person-centered approach aligns very closely with TCM's holistic approach, and the details Hippocratic doctors evaluated are very similar to what TCM practitioners have always considered when examining and treating each patient. Chapter 6 gives you a small window into what you might expect at an appointment with a TCM practitioner.

Healing integratively

Medical products and practices that are not part of standard medical care (Western medicine) are labeled complementary and alternative medicine (CAM), according to the National Institutes of Health and other major health-care systems, such as the United Kingdom's National Health Service. Therefore, TCM is considered CAM among most Western medical professionals. For example, a person can use TCM as a complement to Western medicine, much like a side dish or appetizer to round out the main course. Or a person can use TCM instead of Western medicine, like choosing lasagna instead of fettuccine alfredo.

The term integrative medicine (IM) is catching on as more Western professionals seek a combination of effective approaches for their patients. Dr. Andrew Weil, MD, is a pioneer and proponent of integrative medicine who helped establish it as a specialty. His Center for Integrative Medicine at the University of Arizona offers a range of programs from residency and fellowship to certification for medical doctors, nurses, and other health-care professionals, including acupuncturists. I earned my Integrative Health and Lifestyle (IHeLP) certification from the Center in 2020. The knowledge I gained and continue to access as an IHeLP alumni informs my practice every day.

Because a Western medicine doctor raised me, I greatly appreciate what Western medicine can do. I'm also aware of its shortcomings and risks. Similarly, TCM has enormous benefits (which I hope this book can show you), but it has limitations, too. As a healer, I want people to have access to every healing method available that improves their health and quality of life. By combining traditional and nontraditional treatments, I think integrative medicine moves patients and practitioners toward that goal, bringing the best of all worlds to wellness.

Uncovering TCM's Origins and Principles

For the physicians of ancient Greece, China, and India, a person's health depended on what modern medicine calls *lifestyle* or *preventative* medicine. These ancient physicians believed in keeping illness from becoming a problem in the body. Granted, many health-related issues from 3,000, 1,000, or even 100 years ago differ greatly from modern-day illnesses. But I find it quite interesting that many people continue to use TCM today, which elicits a similar type of curiosity about treating illness.

Observing nature

Every society or culture has developed some kind of response to illness and injury. Historians can certainly debate which came first. The oldest records discovered (on tortoise shells, papyrus rolls, animal skins, fabric, or paper) seem to date back to around 2,000 BCE, but Stone Age healers and their methods existed for a long time before that.

In early societies, healers tried to make sense of why and how things occurred, just as modern physicians do today. But thousands of years ago, they didn't have laboratories or microscopes — they had to observe the world around them with their eyes and other senses. They noted how physical conditions in nature changed when the seasons changed. They saw how wind, rain, cold, and heat affected people. They studied the movement of the sun, moon, and other lights and objects in the sky. Healers meticulously recorded their observations on a variety of materials. In China, ancient healers took copious notes on bamboo slips and silk scrolls as described in the following sections.

Finding evidence in ancient scrolls

Some scholars believe, based on ancient texts, that the two main branches (or components) of TCM — *acupuncture and moxibustion* (burning dried mugwort near points on the body, which I talk about in the section "Discovering TCM beyond the needles," later in this chapter), and *materia medica* (plant, animal, and mineral products used medically) — developed in different parts of China and then somehow merged. As I describe in Chapters 4 and 5, each of the TCM therapies has a very long and interesting history. But you can see the oldest documented proof of TCM's origins in a permanent exhibit at the Hunan Museum in South Central China.

The discovery of the Mawangdui tombs in Changsha, Hunan province, China, in 1973 was like an Indiana Jones moment for not only global archaeology and

Chinese cultural history, but also for TCM. According to a 2024 article in *The Global Times*, workers doing construction drilling for a military hospital project found three tombs. Researchers believe the tombs were built in 168 BCE. The remarkably well-preserved tomb contents included over 50 bamboo and silk scrolls (see Figure 1-1).

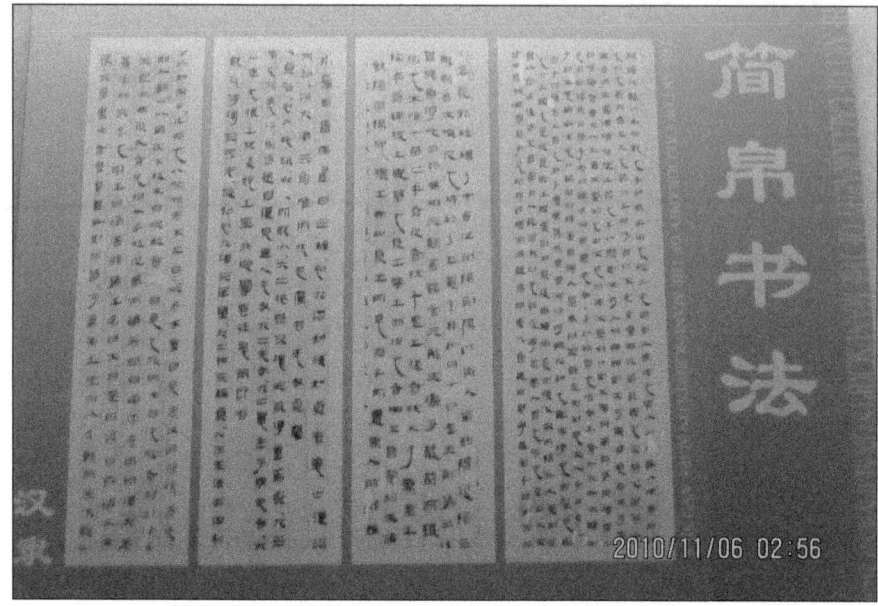

FIGURE 1-1:
Ancient silk scroll unearthed from Mawangdui Han Tomb 3, as preserved in the Hunan Museum.

Huangdan2060/https://commons.wikimedia.org/wiki/File:Mawangdui_Silk_Texts_1.JPG/
Public domain/last accessed on Feb 11, 2026

Among the scrolls found were manuscripts demonstrating the breadth of ancient Chinese medical concepts and techniques. They describe early ideas and theories about how the human body operates and how it gets sick and dies, which are fundamental to TCM.

Of course, Chinese scholars had first dibs on organizing, studying, translating, and discussing these works, but a Japanese research team from Kyoto University published a two-volume collection of translations and essays about them in 1985. I'm not really sticking my neck out too far to say the definitive English translation and discussion of these texts was published in 1998 as *Early Chinese Medical Literature* (Routledge), by Donald J. Harper, PhD, an expert in early Chinese civilization and Centennial Professor of Chinese Studies at the University of Chicago.

The Mawangdui scrolls are the largest collection of medical literature from that time (299–100 BCE). Other tomb discoveries from the same period have expanded our knowledge of early Chinese medicine, including how this knowledge was recorded, shared, and preserved. For more on the Mawangdui discoveries, please see Appendix B.

Seeking spiritual guidance

Although modern medicine operates in the framework of science, medicine evolved from traditional medical practices and theories highly influenced by spiritual, mystical, or religious beliefs. In some cultures, healers were also priests, monks, diviners, shamans, and so on. Whether it was a higher power's punishment or an angry ancestor's curse, many cultures believed that you could reverse or avoid misfortune if you kept the higher powers and ancestors happy — or, at least, not offended.

Some examples of ancient cultures that believed one's health was influenced by the supernatural include:

>> **Mesopotamia:** As far back as 4000 BCE, the societies of Mesopotamia used herbal remedies, prayers, offerings, and rituals to appease the gods and keep evil spirits away.

>> **Egypt:** Ancient Egyptians believed gods, spirits, and demons had a hand in illness. Their earliest medical texts, known as the Pyramid Texts (around 2600 BCE), contained spells, prayers, and incantations for protection. Treatments often involved religious symbols, prayers, and offerings associated with gods and goddesses of healing, such as Sekhmet, the goddess of medicine, or Imhotep, the deified physician and architect of the Step Pyramid of Djoser.

>> **India:** Scholars of *Ayurveda* (India's traditional system of medicine) think that this system has divine origins. This holistic healing knowledge was passed from the Hindu god of creation, Brahma, to Indra, the king of the gods. Indra then shared it with the legendary sage Atreya, who wrote the earliest medical compilations (Vedas) that were later refined by another renowned sage Agnevisha. A key aspect of Ayurvedic practice is spiritual counseling (*satsang*) to help achieve the balance and harmony needed for well-being.

>> **China:** The ancient Chinese early medical framework included magic, astrology, numerology, and *hemerology* (the study of calendars to identify or predict lucky days). As discussed in Chapter 2, TCM concepts tie back to Taoist philosophy, which emphasizes the relationships of opposing yet mutually dependent factors and the interconnectedness of all things.

Focusing on belief concepts

Although modern medicine relies on science for its evidence-based theories and practices, belief has power of its own in the healing process. The evidence in modern medicine is obtained through meticulously constructed clinical trials that are designed to test the safety and efficacy of a new medication or treatment for a certain condition or symptom. To prove that it works well, the medication is compared to a *placebo,* which is a substance designed to have no effect. It has no therapeutic action. One group of testers receives the medication while the other group gets the placebo. The results from the two groups are compared. If the medication is significantly more effective at improving the condition or relieving the symptom than the placebo, it stands a good chance of being approved for production and marketing.

If the placebo group shows improvement despite receiving essentially nothing, this is called a *placebo effect* — the people believed they were given medication, and this belief improved their condition. Professional athletes have certain rituals or routines that they follow that have nothing to do with their physical gifts, mental toughness, or competitive spirit — but they believe that these rituals improve their performance.

In the medical world, I associate the idea of belief with the patient experience and what gives patients faith in practitioners, medicines, treatments, and recommendations. A 2020 joint Healthgrades and Medical Group Management Association study analyzed 8.4 million patient reviews and comments about health-care providers. Over 52 percent of patients indicated they wanted someone who had at least one of the following qualities: compassion, comfort, patience, personality, and bedside manner.

Neurobiology and psychiatry researchers have found that patients who believe that their doctor has good bedside manner are more likely to view their treatment as effective, comply with treatment recommendations, and experience reduced symptoms and better recovery.

The late Herbert Benson, MD, was a Harvard cardiologist who pioneered the field of *mind-body medicine* (which cultivates the interactions among the mind, body, and behavior to promote health). His extensive research, teaching, and publications brought greater awareness to medical professionals and the general public about the effects of spirituality and faith on healing. Benson wrote, "Practicing medicine and conducting medical research, I've learned that invoking beliefs is not only emotionally and spiritually soothing but vitally important to physical health."

Hmm, perhaps TCM also falls in the category of mind-body medicine.

Presenting the TCM Therapies

TCM has deep and ancient roots (which you can read more about in the section "Uncovering TCM's Origins and Principles," earlier in this chapter, with a deeper dive in Chapters 4 and 5). Over the centuries, the trunk has stayed pretty solid, despite efforts to destroy it. During China's Cultural Revolution, from 1966 to 1976, the Chinese government under Mao Zedong attempted to purge all things considered elite (see Chapter 4 for a brief discussion of this attempt), which included TCM.

TCM was deemed elite because it was practiced by physician-scholars who passed their knowledge down through their families or handpicked disciples. This is what I consider *Classical Chinese Medicine* (see the section entitled "Revealing family secrets" in Chapter 4).

Since then, branches of TCM have extended beyond China, offering different approaches, schools of thought, techniques, technologies (such as electricity and lasers), tools, and materials. For this book, I stick with what I learned in my TCM program and the therapies that I can use as a licensed practitioner. (See Chapter 3 for more details about licensing.)

Using acupuncture

Probably the most familiar TCM therapy is *acupuncture,* which involves the insertion of very thin needles at certain points in the body for healing effects. And the most prominent tools of this therapy are the needles. However, acupuncture actually focuses on stimulating specific points on the body. Practitioners most frequently produce stimulation by using needles, but they can also use heat, manual pressure, or electric current. The length and thickness of the needles used and the location of needle insertion depend on the specific issue that the acupuncturist is addressing at the time. You can also apply acupuncture to the scalp and ears.

Different styles of acupuncture get their flavor from the country where they're practiced or reflect new thinking or approaches. For example, Chinese, Korean, and Japanese acupuncture may have the same foundation, but each is distinctly its own practice. Although this book focuses on Chinese acupuncture, here's a summary of the different styles, as explained to me by one of my professors, Dr. Jung Kim, an expert in TCM theory and Korean Saam acupuncture (a style that involves a total of four needles inserted in the hands), who describes the difference in style as a difference in character:

>> **Chinese:** Aggressive, with deep needle insertion and a lot of needle manipulation

>> **Japanese:** Gentle, with shallow needle insertion and little to no needle manipulation

>> **Korean:** Somewhere in between Chinese and Japanese styles, like Korea's geographic position between China and Japan

You can find a more detailed look at acupuncture, its history, and its application in Chapter 4.

Discovering TCM beyond the needles

In addition to acupuncture (discussed in the preceding section and Chapter 4), TCM includes other manual therapies and herbal prescriptions. Here's a brief overview (and you can find more information in Chapter 5):

>> **Moxibustion:** Heat supplied, either directly or indirectly, by burning the herb Artemisia vulgaris (mugwort) over a single acupuncture point, group of points, or area. Its heat penetrates deeply beneath the skin and radiates to deeper tissues like muscles and tendons. Practitioners often use moxibustion to alleviate pain, especially in chronic cases. See Chapter 7 for more information on pain management.

>> **Herbs and/or nutritional supplements:** Include plant, animal, and mineral substances, as well as foods. Whether individual or combined into formulas, TCM prescriptions can facilitate the body's own restorative process and complement other TCM treatments. See Chapter 5 for more details on TCM herbal therapy.

>> **Cupping:** The application of round vacuum cups over an area to enhance blood circulation. Cupping is discussed in Chapter 5.

>> **Gua sha:** Often translated as *scraping,* but you can more accurately describe it as *press-stroking* on lubricated skin by using a smooth-edged tool. Gua sha improves blood circulation, relieves pain, and strengthens the immune system. See Chapter 5 for more on gua sha and Chapter 7 for more on its use in pain relief.

>> **Tui na:** A therapeutic massage developed by classical TCM physicians as a medical therapy in accordance with TCM principles. Practitioners often use it to decrease pain, increase circulation and metabolism, and treat joint disorders. See Chapters 5 and 7 for more details.

>> **Qigong and tai chi:** Movement-based therapies that have multiple physical, mental, and emotional benefits. See Chapter 5 for more information.

Exploring technological components

Two components frequently used during TCM treatment use technology that didn't exist when TCM originated, so I consider them additional features:

>> **Infrared and Teding Diancibo Pu (TDP) lamp therapy:** Warming the skin by using a heat source mounted to an adjustable arm and positioned above the body. Infrared heat helps relieve muscle and joint stiffness and pain. *Teding Diancibo Pu* translates to "special electromagnetic spectrum." This lamp combines infrared heat and a ceramic, mineral-infused plate to improve blood circulation and facilitate healing.

>> **Electrical stimulation (e-stim):** Running a low-level electrical current through the body by attaching small electrodes to inserted acupuncture needles. The concept is very similar to transcutaneous electrical nerve stimulation (TENS), which delivers an electrical current through electrodes attached to pads stuck to the skin. E-stim is more precise than TENS because the needles deliver the current to small, specific parts of the body, while TENS pads cover more surface area.

Deciding to Try TCM

Navigating any health-care system in the modern world can be complicated, to say the least. In my personal experience, it takes persistence, patience, and a fair amount of self-advocacy to get the care that you need. When I'm faced with a challenge or venture into uncharted territory, the better informed I am, the better my chances of success.

In the following sections, I share some thoughts to help your decision-making process as you consider whether TCM is a potential health-care modality.

Figuring out your expectations

If you see TCM as a potential health-care option, start by evaluating why or how you might benefit from it.

Based on what I've heard over 13 years of clinical practice in the United States, some of the reasons may include:

>> Nothing else has worked.

>> I don't want to rely on medication(s).

>> I don't want to have surgery.

>> A friend/family member/coworker suggested I try it.

Although I'm grateful for whatever brings a patient to my door, I recognize that I need to understand the patient's expectations for healing, especially because I provide health care that falls outside of or is other than conventional Western medicine.

If nothing else has worked, why do they think TCM will? If TCM doesn't work, are they out of options? That's a lot of pressure, being the Hail Mary pass of health care. And although drugs and surgery can have pitfalls and risks, TCM has limitations, too. I had a urinary tract infection that a medical doctor remedied by giving me antibiotics faster than I could have by taking a TCM formula and having a session of acupuncture. TCM can't remove a tumor or reconstruct a torn ligament in your knee, but it can surely minimize post-surgical side effects and speed recovery.

I'm always happy when a patient comes to me on the referral of someone they trust. But what works for one person doesn't always work for someone else. TCM treatment is truly tailored to an individual's history and condition, and crafted by the specific training and experience of the practitioner (for more on TCM education and training, see Chapter 3). Ten people can come to me with right shoulder pain, and I can deliver ten different treatments that have varying levels of effectiveness. On the flipside, a patient who has right shoulder pain could go to ten TCM practitioners and get a different treatment each time with varying levels of effectiveness. Because of this variability, I ask new patients to request a referral to another practitioner if they don't get positive results with me within four sessions. More chronic cases can take longer, but if I haven't moved the needle at all on a patient's condition after four treatments, I'm not the right fit. Just like in any good relationship, a little bit of chemistry comes into play.

Knowing your commitment level

When you consider what healing means to you, take into account the level of effort that you, as the patient, can and will put into it. In my welcome letter to new patients, I make it a point to describe my vision of our work together:

> I see this as the beginning of a unique partnership that has been formed with a common goal in mind — your health and well-being. For any partnership to succeed, there needs to be mutual understanding, trust, and effort. As your practitioner partner, I am committed to providing you with the best possible medical care within my scope of practice as an acupuncturist and doctor of Traditional Chinese Medicine. As my patient partner, I ask that you be an active participant in this process to the best of your ability.

IN THIS CHAPTER

» **Considering the theory behind the TCM system**

» **Looking at TCM anatomy**

» **Exploring the 12 channels**

» **Understanding the problems with Qi**

Chapter **2**

Diving into TCM Concepts and Theories

This chapter introduces you to the basic principles and theories that form the foundation of Traditional Chinese Medicine (TCM), based on my understanding and interpretation of the teachings that I received at school, my observation of and dialogue with other practitioners, and my own practice.

One of my professors provided an adage to practice by — the same patient can see ten different TCM practitioners and receive ten different diagnoses and treatments. Just as TCM practitioners individualize treatment for each patient, each TCM practitioner has an individualized knowledge and application of TCM. Accordingly, this chapter (and this book) represents my individual take on TCM.

This chapter offers just a drop in the ocean of thousands of years of collective wisdom, documented in ancient Chinese, interpreted and translated many times over, and taught and adapted all over the world. Here, I give you just the ABCs, do-re-mis, and 1-2-3s of TCM that practitioners in the West start with before embarking on their own paths to help heal people.

Exploring TCM Theory by the Numbers

After my first day in my master's program in TCM, my head was spinning with new concepts and ideas. I grouped this information into a series of numbers to help me organize and recall it for testing. Little did I know then that I'd still be using them all these years later. The following sections explain my groupings.

Explaining the Vital Three

In TCM, three vital or fundamental substances (for lack of a better-translated word) maintain the activities and functions in the human body. TCM refers to the *Vital Three* as Qi or Chi (pronounced "chee"), Blood, and Body Fluid.

Powering the universe with Qi

The most common English translation for *Qi* is *energy.* But in traditional Chinese philosophy and medicine, it's so much more.

The closest term that fits my understanding of Qi is the Force in the *Star Wars* franchise. You can't see it or touch it, but you can feel it. It's everywhere and in everything. It connects all living things and moves. It's strong and weak. Without it, no life can exist. The concept of Qi is rooted in Taoism — one of the religions George Lucas (writer and director of the franchise) referenced to define the Force, as he explained in a 2018 interview.

The Chinese character for Qi, as shown in Figure 2-1, combines two *radicals* (components).

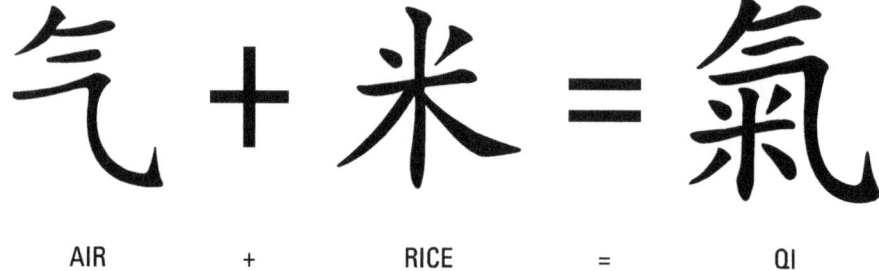

AIR   +   RICE   =   QI

FIGURE 2-1: The traditional Chinese character for Qi.

The first radical, at the top of the character, represents air, which you can translate as *gas, vapor,* or *steam.* The second radical, at the bottom of the character, represents rice (in grain form).

Here's one interpretation that I like: Rice grains heated in water produce steam that changes or transforms the grains into cooked rice. The energy or force required for this to happen is the Qi that resides in each item — the rice grains, water, heat, and steam; the interaction of each item's Qi with that of the other items; and the newly formed collective Qi that results from this interaction. You eat the steamed rice; its Qi enters your body and activates the Qi of your organ systems in a cascade of interactions, like a row of dominoes that fall one after another.

Looking at this process from a Western perspective, I associate air with oxygen and rice with food (and water). The human body needs both to make and maintain the energy or force required to function and live.

The different types and functions of Qi in TCM could fill a book on their own. For current or potential patients, in addition to energy (or force), here are the most important aspects of Qi to know:

>> **Qi moves.** It travels throughout the body along channels or meridians (which I talk about in the section "Following the Major Channels," later in this chapter). It also moves or transports the other vital substances of Blood and Body Fluid, as well as critical components of life, such as oxygen and nutrients.

>> **Qi supports function.** Each organ, tissue, cell, substance, and so on in your body has its own Qi. The condition of this Qi determines how well each one functions and does its job.

>> **Qi acts as both producer and product.** You need Qi to make Qi.

REMEMBER

In TCM theory, you are born with the Qi that you inherit (like genetics) from your parents and ancestors — this is called *pre-natal Qi* or, more poetically, *Essence* (*Jing*, in TCM terms). Like the number of eggs in a woman's ovaries, Essence is finite. It depletes as you age, and it can't be replaced — bummer. You can, however, preserve your Essence with your post-natal Qi. This is the Qi I'm talking about in this section and throughout the book. You replenish, maintain, and strengthen your Qi through food, water, and lifestyle. You damage or weaken your Qi through your choices and your exposure to external and environmental pathogens like viruses and pollution.

>> **Qi problems lead to health problems.** I go into detail on this connection in the section "Identifying the Qi Problem," later in this chapter.

Circulating the Blood

Like Western medicine's definition of blood, TCM's red Blood circulates in the veins and arteries, and delivers important stuff where and when the body needs it.

Western medicine associates blood with transportation — carrying oxygen, nutrients, hormones, waste, and infection fighters (white blood cells) throughout the body. TCM associates Blood with nourishment, moisture, and mental activity. Although TCM describes Blood differently, it has primary functions that are very similar to Western medicine's blood. Both Blood and blood:

>> Feed and sustain the body

>> Keep organs and tissues smooth and supple, instead of dry and stiff, like a lubricant

>> Provide a steady flow of oxygen and nutrients that it carries to allow for proper brain function

Understanding Body Fluid

The vital substance of Body Fluid consolidates all the fluids known in Western medicine into one concept. These fluids may be tested for diagnostic or pathologic purposes. TCM practitioners ask patients about Body Fluid for the same reasons.

While the TCM term is singular, *Body Fluid* includes saliva, tears, urine, digestive juices, and nasal discharge. Like the vital substance Blood (which you can read about in the preceding section), Body Fluid nourishes and moistens. Unlike Blood, Body Fluid acts on or in certain parts of the body: skin, muscles, joints, the brain, and openings such as the mouth, nose, ears, and eyes.

You can think of Body Fluid as "Blood, Jr." because it has a smaller scope of influence.

The Vital Three depend on each other and coordinate with each other to support vital body functions. All three are formed from your intake of food, water, and oxygen. Qi moves Blood and Body Fluid. Qi also helps transform food, water, and oxygen into Blood and Body Fluid. Body Fluid is a component of Blood and vice versa.

Introducing the Five Elements

The Five Elements provide the foundation for how TCM practitioners diagnose and treat health problems in the U.S. Along with the theory of Yin and Yang (which I discuss in the section "Yin and Yang," later in this chapter), the Five Elements theory emerged from observations of natural systems and events made by people and scholars in ancient China. They tried to make sense of why and how things occurred, just as modern scientists do today. But 2,000-plus years ago, they didn't have a controlled laboratory for research or microscopes to observe things too small for the human eye to see on its own. They observed the land and sky by using their eyes and other senses.

In their observations, the ancient Chinese noticed five natural/raw materials essential to daily living: Earth, Metal, Water, Wood, and Fire. They noted the interactions of these elements, as well as their relationships and dependencies. Over centuries, the theory evolved as an overarching framework and expanded to explain other natural phenomena, such as the human body.

Ancient Chinese philosophers and physicians used the Five Elements as a classification system to organize what they observed and interpreted into one of the Five Elements' categories — Earth, Metal, Water, Wood, and Fire.

I can't unpack thousands of years of reasoning and records in this book, but in the following sections, I do share some of the items in each Five Elements category that are relevant to TCM diagnosis and treatment.

Defining the Five Elements' categories

For the purposes of diagnosis and treatment, TCM associates certain items with each of the Five Elements categories. The items that fall into each Element category include specific organs, senses, tissues, body fluids, emotions, actions/functions, environmental pathogens (referred to as *external evils*, environmental influences that attack the body and cause illness), seasons, colors, and flavors/tastes. I discuss the organs in more detail in the section "Examining TCM anatomy," later in this chapter.

Here's a summary of each Five Elements category:

>> **Earth:** You plant seeds in the earth, where they are fed and sheltered until they grow into whatever they're meant to become. You can also shape and harden earth to become bricks for buildings or containers for storing.

>> **Metal:** Humans use metal for everything from coins and jewelry to pots and pitchforks to wire and knives. Metal is durable, yet it's also pliable or bendable. Metal conducts heat and electricity. Metal can be solid or liquid.

>> **Water:** All living things need water. Our planet is mostly water. Our bodies are mostly water. Water cools, cleans, and carries.

>> **Wood:** People use wood to build houses and furniture, to create paper, and as a source of fuel. Wood is also strong, flexible, and renewable.

>> **Fire:** Fire can destroy, but Fire also generates heat and stimulates growth and transformation.

Table 2-1 breaks down the items associated with each of the Five Elements categories. For example, you can see in the first row of the table that the organs associated with the Earth element are the spleen and stomach. The next section describes how TCM practitioners understand the relationships among the Five Elements and the items associated with them.

TABLE 2-1 **Five Elements Categories and Associated Items**

Associated Items	Earth	Metal	Water	Wood	Fire
Organs	Spleen and stomach	Lungs and large intestine	Kidneys and urinary bladder	Liver and gallbladder	Heart and pericardium/ small intestine and san jiao
Sense	Mouth (taste)	Nose (smell)	Ear (hearing)	Eye (sight)	Tongue (taste)
Body tissues and fluids	Muscle and thin, watery saliva	Skin, hair, and nasal discharge	Bone and thick, sticky saliva	Tendons and tears	Vessels and sweat
Emotion	Worry	Grief or sadness	Fear	Anger	Joy
Actions/ functions	Transforming and transporting, receiving, and holding/containing	Dispersing and descending	Storing, moistening, flowing downwards	Growing, ascending, and flourishing	Expanding, evaporating, and flaring
Environmental pathogen	Dampness	Dryness	Cold	Wind	Heat
Season	Late summer	Autumn	Winter	Spring	Summer
Color	Yellow	White	Black	Green	Red
Flavor/taste	Sweet	Acrid (bitter)	Salty	Sour	Aromatic (spicy)

Understanding the Five Elements' relationships

As in nature, the Five Elements of Earth, Metal, Water, Wood, and Fire interact with each other in the human body in various ways.

>> Sometimes, they cooperate.

>> Sometimes, they oppose.

>> Sometimes, they encourage and support.

>> Sometimes, they drain and diminish.

>> Sometimes, they feed into each other in a generative cycle.

>> Sometimes, they limit or constrain in a counteractive cycle.

As with many types of relationships, you may experience both smooth sailing and stormy seas when it comes to the relationships of the Five Elements. When family members or business partners each pull their weight and work as a harmonious unit, life is good. When someone slacks off, undermines the work of others, or micromanages their activities, life isn't so good.

The theory of the Five Elements basically involves a series of coordinated, inter-dependent relationships that allow all things in the universe to function and thrive. Applied to the human body, the health of these relationships determines the health of a person. If you can heal these relationships, then you can heal a person.

Here's the tricky part to understand. These relationships exist interdependently within the *Five Elements cycle.* When any one of the Five Elements' relationships changes, a cascade of interactions occurs that disrupts the entire cycle and affects the relationships among the other Five Elements.

No wonder we humans rarely operate in perfect harmony! Like a car engine, we require repair and maintenance to keep this Five Elements cycle running smoothly. In TCM, practitioners identify the main relationship for a specific health condition, and then use acupuncture, herbs, and other treatments to address that relationship.

As described in the Mawangdui scrolls (see Chapter 1), how the Five Elements relate to each other and interact indicates health or illness in the body. TCM text-book translations refer to these relationships or interactions as:

>> Promoting (supporting)

>> Interacting (controlling or restraining)

>> Counteracting (taking advantage of)

>> Overacting (overcontrolling or overbearing)

In the following sections, I provide examples to explain the Five Elements' relationships and interactions, which I characterize as a family dynamic.

REMEMBER

Each Five Elements relationship represents the balance or the imbalance that affects health and illness. TCM practitioners reference these relationships to evaluate a patient's signs and symptoms to determine a diagnosis and treatment plan.

PROMOTING: THE SUPPORTIVE RELATIONSHIP

Figure 2-2 shows the Five Elements cycle in its normal, clockwise pattern. Each element provides support to the next element in the cycle, like a parent to a child. So, the parent *promotes* the child. TCM practitioners consider this relationship normal and beneficial, like a parent who provides the sustenance and guidance for a child to thrive.

For example, when Wood promotes Fire, the liver (see "Examining TCM Anatomy," later in this chapter) supports the heart — storing blood and regulating its volume during circulation. Clinically, the *promoting* relationship maintains normal blood pressure and blood coagulation.

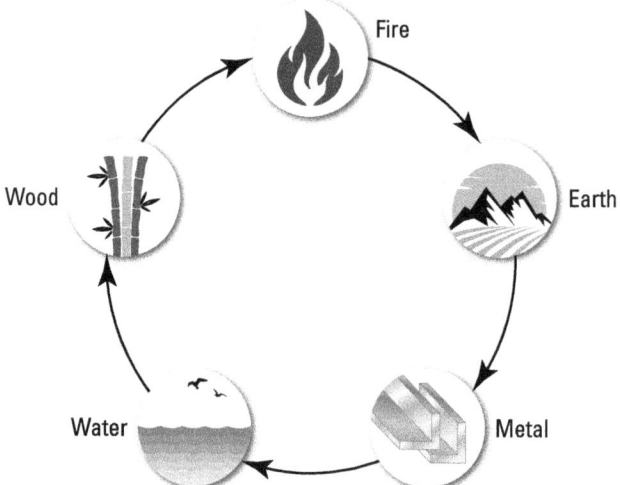

FIGURE 2-2:
Each element *promotes* (supports) the next element.

INTERACTING: THE CONTROLLING RELATIONSHIP

In the Five Elements relationship known as *interacting* (a positive relationship in the cycle, just like the promoting cycle, discussed in the preceding section), each element helps control the element that appears two places clockwise in the cycle, as illustrated in Figure 2-3. Think of this relationship like a grandparent watching out for their grandchild. The grandparent helps to reinforce both parental support and limits so that the child is still nurtured but isn't an undisciplined brat.

When Wood interacts with Earth, as shown in Figure 2-3, the liver (see "Examining TCM Anatomy," later in this chapter) controls or influences the spleen's function of transforming food into Qi and transporting it throughout the body. In TCM theory, one of the key functions of the liver is to "maintain the free flow of Qi." So, clinically, this *interacting* relationship results in easy digestion and nutrient distribution.

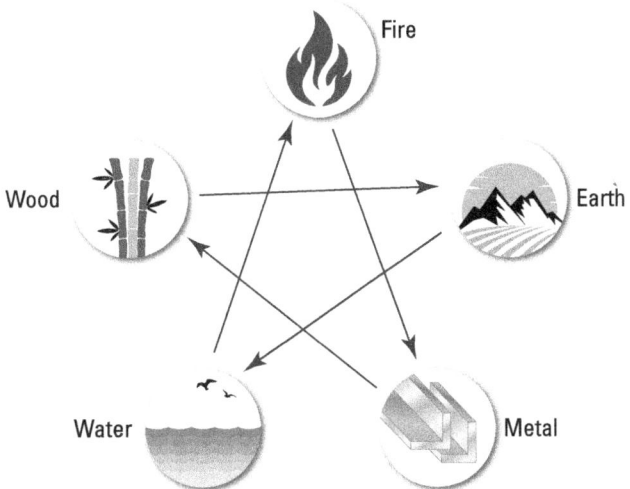

FIGURE 2-3:
Each element
interacts with
(controls)
another element.

REMEMBER

In a healthy Five Elements system, according to ancient Chinese practitioners, the parent supports the child, and the grandparent keeps the child from being spoiled and unruly. The interacting relationship plays out normally if the give-and-take between the elements is just right.

COUNTERACTING: THE OPPORTUNISTIC RELATIONSHIP

The *counteracting* relationship in the Five Elements cycle is a negative interaction between the same two elements in an *interacting* relationship (see the preceding section). Counteracting only occurs when the grandparent element is weak. The grandchild element takes advantage of this weakness and counteracts the grandparent element's control.

In my initial take on this relationship, I saw it as combative, like a kid talking back or being deliberately defiant. Over time, I realized this relationship more closely resembles exploitation, like taking more than you need or slacking off on your responsibilities.

When Earth counteracts Wood, as shown in Figure 2-4, the liver (see "Describing the organs," later in this chapter) is in a weakened condition and unable to adequately facilitate the free flow of Qi. The spleen takes this opportunity to get lazy and doesn't transform nutrients efficiently or transport them in a timely manner. Clinically, this *counteracting* relationship can cause bloating, constipation, or even pain.

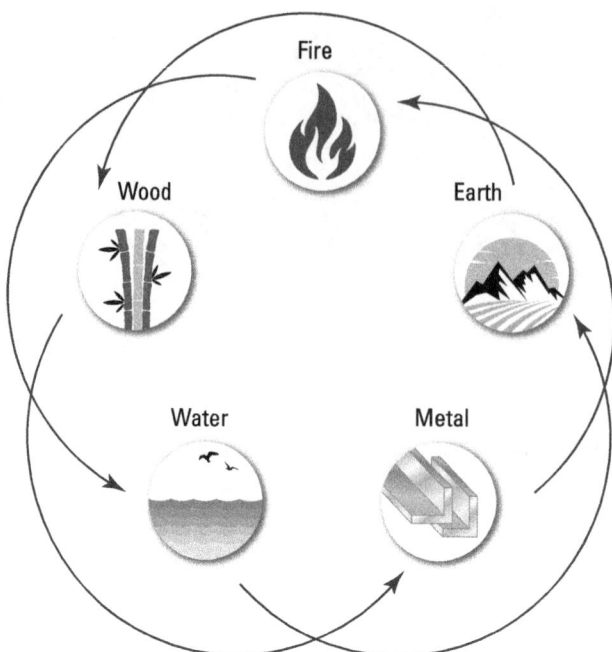

OVERACTING: THE OVERBEARING RELATIONSHIP

The *overacting* relationship occurs between the same two elements as the *interacting* relationship (see section above). However, in this unfavorable situation, the grandparent element is overwhelming the grandchild element with attention or withholding it.

In Figure 2-5, the *overacting* relationship is identical to Figure 2-3, so it's not visually different. But when Wood overacts on Earth, the liver (see "Examining TCM Anatomy," later in this chapter) is not maintaining the free flow of Qi, and the spleen is less able to manage the transformation and transportation of nutrients and Qi. Clinically, this *overacting* relationship can also cause bloating, constipation, or even pain.

The *counteracting* and *overacting* relationships in the Five Elements cycle (see preceding section) work at cross purposes, so the cycle breaks down. These two unhealthy relationships occur only when the parent element — promoting (discussed in the section "Promoting: The supportive relationship," earlier in this chapter) — or the grandparent element — interacting (see "Interacting: The controlling relationship," earlier in this chapter) — is too weak to withstand the counteracting or overacting of the child or grandchild element.

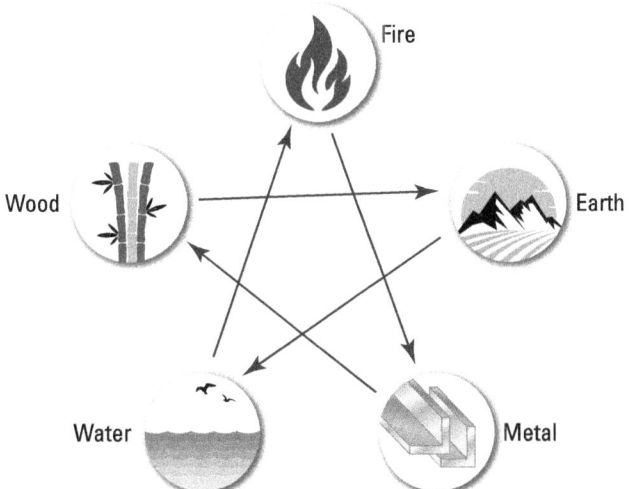

FIGURE 2-5:
Each element
can *overact*
(overwhelm)
another element.

**AUTHOR
SAYS**

At first, I wondered why the Five Elements cycle included only one type of parent–child relationship. You can certainly find parents who don't discipline their children, children who take every opportunity to get the better of their parents, and parents who are overbearing with their children. My interpretation is that the early TCM practitioners most consistently observed these cycle dynamics, and the English translation in our texts is an approximation of ancient Chinese terms.

Maintaining the Eight Balances

In the Chinese philosophy of Taoism and its TCM application, the idea of balance doesn't relate to two sides of a scale being even. It's about two somewhat opposing, complementary, interdependent forces that must exist together to exist at all.

In simple terms, Taoism is a way to live in harmony or balance with the universe and its unifying energy — Qi (for more on this philosophy/religion, I refer you to its primary text, *Tao Te Ching*, by Lao Tze). As discussed in the earlier section on the Vital Three ("Explaining the Vital Three"), Qi is central to TCM theory and practice.

In addition to the Five Elements, the novice practitioner learns to recognize and evaluate four pairs of principles, known as the *Eight Balances:*

- » Yin or Yang

- » Hot or cold

- » Deficiency or excess

- » Exterior or interior

TAOISM: THE GUIDING PHILOSOPHY OF TCM

As I note in Chapter 1, every culture developed a response to illness — their medicine — that reflected their people's beliefs and interpretations of how the world worked and their place in it. For the early Chinese people and their healers, TCM was the medical expression of the Taoist worldview.

TECHNICAL STUFF

How dominant or prevalent one of the pair is compared to the other can uncover clues related to pathogenesis and diagnosis, and a subsequent treatment plan. The root of Taoism and TCM revolves around the theory of Yin and Yang. Yin and Yang are the two opposing, complementary, interdependent forces responsible for everything in the universe. Taoist theory classifies all things based on this original pair.

Yin and Yang

Most people think of Yin and Yang as opposites, like slow and fast, dark and light, and so on. And you may know the famous symbol, called the *Taiji*, representing their unique partnership (see Figure 2-6). The black side is Yin, which includes a spot of white (Yang), and the white side is Yang with a spot of black (Yin).

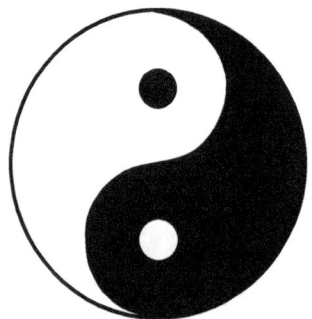

FIGURE 2-6:
The black side is Yin, and the white side is Yang.

As mentioned earlier, Yin and Yang make up the overarching framework for TCM theory, the fundamental nature of all things, as understood by early philosophers, scientists, and healers — heaven and Earth, man and woman, good and evil, and so on. But, as the symbol shows, these duos aren't opposites. Instead of being starkly divided by a straight line, they weave together. Without one side, the symbol ceases to have any meaning or purpose at all. They complete each other.

Because each side contains a seed of its opposite, as the saying goes, it's not all black and white. And all things are relative: You may find something cold that doesn't feel cold to me. An Olympic sprinter runs fast, and in comparison, I run slowly. But put me up against a turtle, and I become the fast one!

Table 2-2 provides some examples to further illustrate Yin-Yang theory. Consider how the world would change if one or the other didn't exist.

TABLE 2-2

Examples of Yin-Yang Duos

Yin	Yang
Down	Up
Earth	Sky
Moon	Sun
Night	Day
Water	Fire
Cold	Hot
Stillness	Movement
Descending	Ascending
Internal	External
Structure/Substance (Noun)	Function (Verb)

TCM applies Yin-Yang theory in the following ways:

>> **Body structure/organization:** The human body is a miraculous, integrated assembly of parts that works seamlessly as a whole entity (except when it gets sick or damaged). Using Yin-Yang theory, the early TCM practitioners divided each of these parts into Yin and Yang features, as shown in Figure 2-7.

The upper half of the body is Yang, and the lower half is Yin. The outside (or surface) of the body is Yang, and the inside (or under the surface of the skin) is Yin. The arms and legs are Yang, and the torso/trunk is Yin. In addition, each organ in the body has Yin and Yang properties.

>> **Body functions:** The body at work reflects the interdependence of Yin and Yang. As Table 2-2 illustrates, Yin is stability (stillness and structure), while Yang is activity (movement and function). Yin is the playing field, and Yang is the activity (running, throwing, or kicking, for example) that takes place on it.

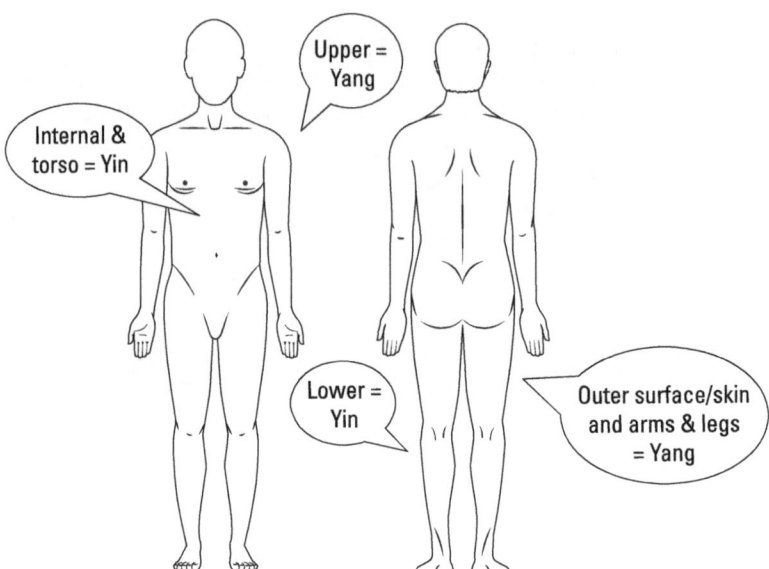

FIGURE 2-7:
Yin–Yang
correspondences
in body structure.

REMEMBER

>> **Body pathology:** Very simply, illness or disease occurs when Yin and Yang aren't balanced.

>> **Diagnosis and treatment:** To solve the mystery of an illness, a TCM practitioner can analyze the illness by examining the Yin and Yang characteristics of the signs and symptoms to determine what's wrong and how to fix it.

Cold and hot

Cold and hot (also referred to as *heat*) describe the basic nature or character of an illness. A patient wants extra blankets in a 78-degree room, has no fever, but does have cold hands and a pale face. These characteristics are cold *signs* (things visible to an outside observer) and cold *symptoms* (things felt and reported by the patient). Hot signs and symptoms could include removing a coat in a 58-degree room and having a fever, sweaty hands, and a red face.

In the Yin-Yang framework, cold signs and symptoms indicate a Yin condition, while hot signs and symptoms point to a Yang one.

Deficiency and excess

The principles of deficiency and excess describe the state of the body's defenses in relation to the pathogens attacking it. Deficiency (also known as *deficient*) indicates the weakness and scarcity of any of the Vital Three — Qi, Blood, Body

Fluid (see the section "Explaining Qi and the Vital Three," earlier in this chapter) — and Yin and/or Yang (discussed in the section "Yin and Yang," earlier in this chapter).

Excess (also known as *excessive*) indicates the strength and overabundance of external and internal pathogens compared to the strength and sufficiency of the Vital Three, and Yin and Yang.

This pair of principles relates to the Five Elements cycle discussed in the preceding section. For example, the lungs in TCM (see "Examining TCM Anatomy," later in this chapter) maintain the body's defenses against external pathogens like a virus. If your Lung Qi is deficient, you will be more likely to catch a cold if you happen to be out at night without a coat. But you can still catch a cold with adequate Lung Qi if you get caught in the excessive cold of a snowstorm.

Deficiency is too little, *excess* is too much, and just enough is just right.

Exterior and interior

Exterior and interior refer to the location of the illness and where it came from. An *exterior* (external) illness tends to show up on the more shallow or external areas of the body and comes from outside the body, such as catching a cold. An *interior* (internal) illness resides deeper in the body yet still manifests symptoms like a fever on the outside, and develops from pathogens building up inside, like when a cold moves into the lungs and becomes pneumonia.

Usually, exterior and interior also indicate the duration of a condition. A cold comes on quickly and normally runs its course in a week, while pneumonia develops over time and can take quite a while to recover from.

REMEMBER

TCM theory is extremely complex, but for me, the two words at its core are *relationships* and *balance*.

Examining TCM Anatomy

All medical approaches recognize that the human body is constructed of the same materials (for example, bones and flesh) and in the same general structure (including a head, torso, arms, and legs), and is powered by the same organs and systems (heart, lungs, circulatory, respiratory, and so on).

However, TCM classifies and characterizes human anatomy by the theories of Yin-Yang and the Five Elements. TCM recognizes three groups of internal organs:

>> **Zang:** Yin organs

- Heart
- Kidneys
- Liver
- Lungs
- Pericardium
- Spleen

>> **Fu:** Yang organs

- Gallbladder
- Large intestine
- Small intestine
- Stomach
- San Jiao (Triple Burner)

>> **Extraordinary Fu:** Neither Yin nor Yang, but organs nonetheless

- Bones
- Brain
- Marrow
- Uterus
- Vessels

To keep things as simple as possible, the following sections focus on each of the organ groups listed above — Zang, Fu, and Extraordinary Fu (Extra Fu, for short). Each organ is associated with one of the Five Elements (see the section "Introducing the Five Elements," earlier in this chapter), and each has its own Qi (which I talk about in the section "Qi," earlier in this chapter).

Like a car, the mechanics and structure of the human body are vast and intricate. What follows is a peek under the hood.

Although TCM theory represents each of the major organs that you know, they have partners, associations, functions, and traits that Western medicine doesn't recognize. A few organs that Western medicine considers minor or conceptually nonexistent act as major players in TCM.

As noted in Table 2-2, earlier in this chapter, Yin is structure, and Yang is function. Accordingly, the Zang (Yin) organs are containers that produce and store the Vital Three (see the section "Explaining Qi and the Vital Three," earlier in this chapter), among other things. The Fu (Yang) organs are conduits that receive and digest food and discard waste. The Extra Fu are not categorized as Yin or Yang or included in Five Element theory. (I was never taught why, nor did I think to ask.)

In the eleventh chapter of *Basic Questions (Su Wen)* (see the "Getting Blood with a Stone: Ancient Origins" section of Chapter 4), the zang organs are described as storing "pure essential qi" without draining it off, and therefore, they can be constantly replenished. The six Fu organs are described as moving water and food without storing them, and for this reason, they have the potential of receiving too much, but they cannot be filled up because their contents are steadily being moved out.

Earth: Spleen and stomach

The spleen and stomach are paired under the Earth sign. The spleen:

>> Is located in the middle of the body, below the diaphragm

>> Relates to worry and overthinking

>> Transports and transforms blood

>> Maintains blood circulation

>> Nourishes/dominates muscles and limbs

AUTHOR
SAYS

I think that the spleen, as discussed in TCM, actually represents multiple smaller organs and glands, like the pancreas, that affect your immune, digestive, and endocrine (hormone) systems.

The stomach:

>> Is located in the middle of the body between the esophagus and the small intestine.

>> Receives, digests, and decomposes food and water/liquids.

>> Sends waste down to the small intestine. (Flip to the section "Fire: Heart and small intestine," later in this chapter, for discussion of the small intestine.)

Metal: Lungs and large intestine

The lungs and large intestine are associated with the element Metal in TCM. The lungs:

>> Are located in the mid to upper body/chest

>> Relate to grief and/or sadness

>> Control Qi movement and breathing

>> Spread Qi and Body Fluid to warm and moisten skin and hair

>> Descends Qi and Body Fluid to regulate water circulation and elimination

The large intestine:

>> Is located in the abdomen, below the lungs and stomach. It connects to the small intestine at the top and the anus at the bottom

>> Receives waste from the small intestine

>> Absorbs any fluid content and eliminates the remaining solid waste

Water: Kidneys and urinary bladder

TCM associates the kidneys and urinary bladder with the element Water. The kidneys:

>> Are located near your lower back, on both sides of the spine

>> Relate to fear and courage

>> Control the reproductive process and organs, and the development and growth of the body

>> Regulate how the body retains, distributes, and discharges water

>> Supports inhalation

>> Determines bone and marrow health

>> Influences the brain

AUTHOR SAYS

In TCM, the kidneys are the source and keeper of Essence (see the discussion on post-natal Qi in the section entitled "Powering the universe with Qi," earlier in this chapter). Essence is derived from the Qi that your parents and ancestors gave you or your genetic constitution. Essence is a subcategory of Qi that can't be reproduced or replenished. Whatever you have when you're born is all that you can ever have, and you can use it up by overworking (or under-resting), having children, or using drugs or other substances. Bummer.

The urinary bladder:

>> Is located in the lower abdomen, below the kidneys

>> Filters and temporarily stores urine

>> Eliminates urine

Wood: Liver and gallbladder

The liver and gallbladder are associated with the Wood element. The liver:

>> Is located in the middle of the body on the right side, protected by the lower ribs

>> Relates to anger and irritability

>> Stores blood

>> Maintains the free flow of Qi

>> Influences the tendons

The gallbladder:

>> Is attached to the bottom of the liver

>> Stores bile and sends it to the intestines to aid digestion

>> Supports the free flow of Qi

>> Relates to emotional stability

Fire: Heart and small intestine

The heart and small intestine are the organs associated with the element Fire. The heart:

>> Is located in the upper-middle body, on the left side of the chest

>> Relates to joy and happiness

>> Controls mental activity, thoughts, and emotions

>> Dominates the blood and its vessels; therefore, it controls blood circulation and containment (keeping blood in the vessels)

The small intestine:

>> Is located in the abdomen, connecting to the stomach above and the large intestine below

>> Receives and further digests food from the stomach

>> Separates liquids from solids — absorbing important substances and sending the remaining liquid waste to the urinary bladder (discussed in the section, "Water: Kidneys and urinary bladder," earlier in this chapter) and the solid waste to the large intestine (see the section "Metal: Lungs and large intestine," earlier in this chapter)

Fire: Pericardium and San Jiao

In TCM, the pericardium is known as "xin bao luo," which loosely means "heart wrapping." It's not listed formally as a Zang organ, but because it surrounds the heart, it's associated with the Fire element. The pericardium:

>> Covers the heart (like bubble wrap)

>> Protects the heart from external pathogens and jostling in the chest space

The triple burner (translated from *san jiao*) is a single Fu organ that has three parts, but no physical form. It is a TCM concept that the ancient practitioners conceived to delineate the upper, middle, and lower sections of the body. Each section regulates the Qi of certain organs located there and helps Qi and Body Fluid move throughout the body like an irrigation system.

The upper burner:

>> Is associated with the heart and lungs

>> Coordinates with the heart and lungs to disperse and distribute Qi to the body

The middle burner:

>> Is associated with the spleen and stomach

>> Coordinates with the spleen and stomach to digest and transform food and water into nutrients and Qi

The lower burner:

>> Is associated with the kidneys, urinary bladder, and large intestine

>> Coordinates with these organs to separate waste fluids and solids and eliminate them from the body

Extraordinary Fu

In addition to the Yin organs (Zang) and Yang organs (Fu), TCM theory identifies several Extraordinary Fu organs: the bones, brain, marrow, uterus, and vessels. The ancient physicians didn't classify these organs in the Five Elements categories because they believed these organs served all of the body and exhibited both Yin and Yang aspects. For instance, the Extraordinary Fu are structured like Yang organs (conduits), but they function like Yin organs (containers).

The bones and marrow are associated with the kidneys and the Water element, and the vessels are associated with the heart and the Fire element.

The brain and the uterus are not associated with any Zang or Fu organ, nor with any element. However, each is associated with a channel or pathway that circulates Qi and Blood, and is used to locate points for treatment (see the next section "Following the Major Channels"). The brain and uterus are described here:

The brain:

>> Is located in the head

>> Controls mental activities such as memory, sight, smell, sound, and speech

>> Relates to physical strength and stamina

TECHNICAL STUFF

When developing TCM theory, the ancient physicians didn't have the advantage of modern technology or techniques to gain a full understanding of the brain. Yet, they did consider the brain to be overrated as the "nucleus" of the body. Instead, the ancient physicians truly embraced the concept of the "body-mind," understanding that consciousness exists in all of our organs, as well as within our blood.

The uterus:

>> Is located in the lower abdomen, behind the urinary bladder

>> Produces menstruation

>> Manages pregnancy

>> Protects and supports the fetus

Discussing the Extraordinary Fu organs further is like taking apart an engine and putting it back together — far more effort and time than you or I may want to invest right now.

Following the Major Channels

The ancient physicians organized the points used in TCM treatment along *channels* (pathways through which Qi and Blood circulate; also known as *meridians*) and *collaterals* (supplemental channels), which remind me of rivers and tributaries. Each channel is associated with one of the 12 Yin organs (Zang) and Yang organs (Fu), plus the two Extraordinary Fu organs described in the preceding section (the brain and uterus).

Humans develop towns and cities along rivers, and agricultural regions abound near rivers and streams. And in the same way that rivers and tributaries transport, connect, and sustain continents and countries, channels and collaterals do the same for the human body.

REMEMBER

Channels and collaterals connect the interior to the exterior, the top to the bottom, and all the organs and tissues in between. The channels run vertically (north–south, like the odd-numbered U.S. interstate highways), and the collaterals branch off of the channels horizontally (east–west, like the even-numbered U.S. interstates). The early practitioners who codified TCM theory believed Qi moved along the channels in a fixed order. (I still don't know where this order comes from; perhaps another 10 years of practice will offer enlightenment.)

Channel functions

As an intricate connected network, the body's channels (and their collaterals) play a significant role in three areas: *physiology* (how a living organism, or a part of one, functions), *pathology* (how illness develops to cause malfunctions), and *prevention or treatment* (how to keep an illness from developing or help to resolve it):

>> **Physiology:** When the body is working normally, the channel system

 • Transports Qi and Blood to moisten and nourish the entire body

 • Regulates and balances Yin and Yang to maintain normal physiological activities and protect the body from external pathogens

>> **Pathology:** When something goes wrong, the channel system

- Transfers pathogens from the exterior to the interior (see the section, "Maintaining the Eight Balances," earlier in this chapter), worsening a condition

- Reflects signs and symptoms to indicate which associated organ(s) are affected

>> **Prevention and treatment:** To prevent and treat a condition, the channel system

- Transmits the sensations and effects of acupuncture to the appropriate organ(s)

- Regulates and/or restores the balance of deficiency and excess (discussed in the section "Maintaining the Eight Balances," earlier in this chapter) to prevent and/or treat the condition

Channel mapping

To give you a sense of the channel pathways (shown in Figure 2-8), I briefly describe each one in the following list:

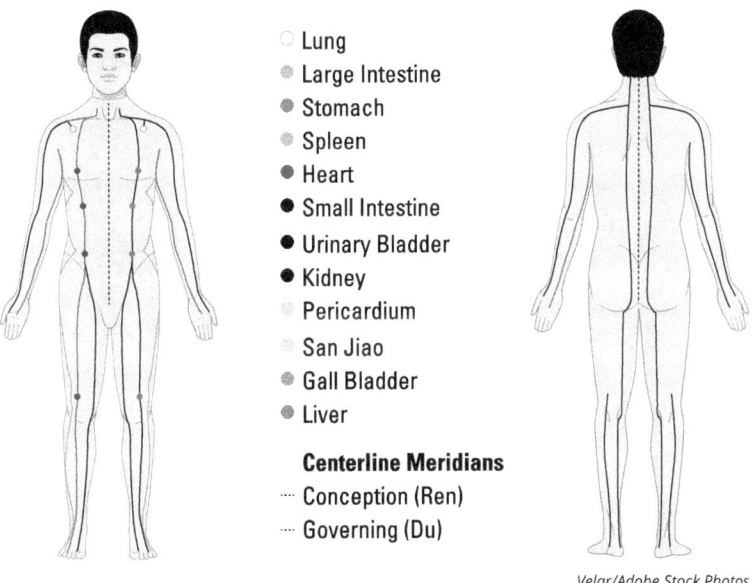

- Lung
- Large Intestine
- Stomach
- Spleen
- Heart
- Small Intestine
- Urinary Bladder
- Kidney
- Pericardium
- San Jiao
- Gall Bladder
- Liver

Centerline Meridians
··· Conception (Ren)
··· Governing (Du)

FIGURE 2-8: The channel pathways.

Velar/Adobe Stock Photos

>> **The Lung channel:** Starts in the belly area, moves down to the large intestine, makes its way up to the lungs, runs down each arm, and ends at the thumb.

- » **The Large Intestine channel:** Starts at the tip of the index (second) finger, runs up the arm to the shoulder, scoots over to the base of the neck, moves down past the lungs, and ends in the large intestine. At the shoulder, a branch winds up the neck and ends on either side of the nose.

- » **The Stomach channel:** Starts at the side of the nose, moves up the jawline to the hairline, comes down the neck through the chest and abdomen, where it meets the spleen, runs down the outer leg, and ends at the tip of the second toe.

- » **The Spleen channel:** Starts at the tip of the big toe, runs up the inner side of the leg, and goes up through the abdomen, where it meets the stomach, enters the throat, and ends in the tongue.

- » **The Heart channel:** Starts in the heart, connects to the other organs in its vicinity, and moves down to the small intestine. From the chest, a small branch goes up to connect with the eyes, and the main branch emerges from the armpit and runs down the arm, ending at the tip of the pinkie (fifth) finger.

- » **The Small Intestine channel:** Starts at the tip of the pinkie, runs up the back of the arm to the shoulder, zigzags across and over the back of the shoulder, connects with the heart, and moves down to the stomach and into the small intestine. At the shoulder, a small branch goes up the side of the neck past the cheek into the ear.

- » **The Urinary Bladder channel:** Starts beside the inner corner of the eye, travels up and over the top of the head to connect with the brain, runs down both sides of the spine to the low back, meets the kidneys and the urinary bladder, runs down the buttock and back of the leg, and ends at the tip of the little toe.

- » **The Kidney channel:** Starts at the little toe, crosses under the arch, runs along the inner side of the foot and up the inner leg to the spine, meets the urinary bladder and the kidneys, climbs up the abdomen and chest through the lungs and throat, and ends at the root of the tongue.

- » **The Pericardium channel:** Starts in the chest and pericardium and descends through the chest and abdomen to connect with the three sections of the San Jiao — upper, middle, and lower. A branch from the chest runs down the arm between the Heart and Lung channels and ends at the tip of the middle finger.

- » **The San Jiao channel:** Starts at the tip of the ring finger, runs up the arm and over the shoulder to meet the pericardium, and descends to connect with all three sections — upper, middle, and lower. From the chest, a branch goes up the side of the neck and winds around the ear to the hairline, turns down to the cheek, and ends under the eye socket.

» **The Gallbladder channel:** Starts at the outer corner of the eye, goes up the side of the head near the temple, does a U-turn at the forehead, goes down and around behind the ear to the neck, moves down the side of the chest and abdomen to connect with the liver and gallbladder, zigs forward to the groin area, zags back to the hip, and runs down the outer leg to end at the big toe.

» **The Liver channel:** Starts at the big toe, moves up the top of the foot, runs up the inner leg to the groin, curves around the genitals and up around the stomach to connect with the liver and gallbladder, continues up the neck and past the eye area to the forehead, and connects with other channels at the top of the head. A branch from the liver moves up to the lungs, where the cycle starts again.

» **The Du channel:** Starts in the pelvis, runs up the spine to the base of the neck, enters the brain, goes up to the top of the head, comes down the middle of the forehead, and ends at the upper lip.

Du translates to *governing* or *commanding*. The Du channel is associated with the Extraordinary Fu organ of the brain. It connects with all the Yang organ channels and therefore governs or influences them.

» **The Ren channel:** Starts in the pelvis, runs up the midline of the front of the body from the genital area to the chin, and ends under the eye.

Ren translates to *fostering* or *conceiving*. The Ren channel is associated with the Extraordinary Fu organ of the Uterus. It connects with all the Yin organ meridians and therefore fosters them to support conception and reproduction.

ADDITIONAL CHANNELS AND COLLATERALS

The Du and Ren channels are two of what are known as the eight extra channels. Essentially, these extra channels link and weave the 12 primary channels to facilitate the movement of the Vital Three and support the functions of all the organs. The extra channels can serve as reservoirs to supply the primary channels with the Vital Three if those channels run low. They can also drain off excess Body Fluid to prevent flooding that could overwhelm the system.

Finding and using hundreds of channel points

To activate the Qi of the organ systems, TCM practitioners perform acupuncture (or acupressure), stimulation with a needle (or manual pressure), at specific points on the channel pathways. These points bring the Qi of the organs to the surface of the body, and stimulating the Qi found at these points restores balance, and thereby, maintains or recovers health.

The two Chinese characters combined to signify an *acupuncture point* are translated as *transportation* and *hole* (see Figure 2-9). Centuries of practice and observation by countless practitioners have not only identified the precise location of these transportation holes, but also their individual and combined effects. Furthermore, each point has a specific name that reflects its location and/or function.

FIGURE 2-9: Chinese characters for an acupuncture point.

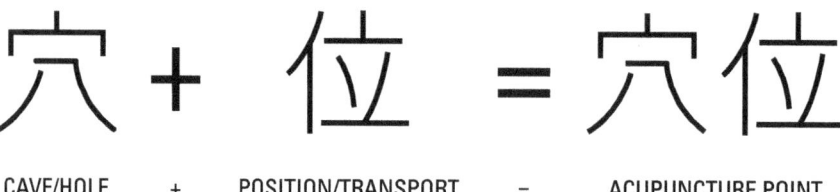

穴 + 位 = 穴位

CAVE/HOLE + POSITION/TRANSPORT = ACUPUNCTURE POINT

The points taught to modern TCM practitioners encompass those of the 14 channels presented in the preceding section, as well as extra points that are not located on any channel. The extra points typically help to address a local issue; for example, an extra point on the shoulder helps with shoulder stiffness. In total, TCM practitioners get familiar with well over 360 individual points on the body in preparation for licensure. (But based on my experience to date, I use less than 20 percent of them in clinical practice.)

Table 2-3 shows how many points each of the 14 major channels contains.

TABLE 2-3

Number of Points by Channel

Channel	Total Points
Lung	11
Large intestine	20
Stomach	45
Spleen	21
Heart	9

Channel	Total Points
Small intestine	19
Urinary bladder	67
Kidney	27
Pericardium	9
San Jiao (triple burner)	23
Gallbladder	44
Liver	14
Ren	24
Du	28
Extra points	48
TOTAL	381

Identifying the Qi Problem

Based on TCM theory, when Yin and Yang are balanced and functioning in harmony, all is well in the universe and in our bodies. Unfortunately, as the early thinkers observed and most of us can acknowledge, balance is hard to achieve and nearly impossible to maintain. We all catch a cold at some point in our lives (and I wish that was the worst of it).

Despite TCM's complexity, its perspective on health is astonishingly simple — imbalance leads to illness. This imbalance can occur in multiple ways, but from my perspective, you can identify all these imbalances as a problem with Qi.

At a very basic level, TCM practitioners try to answer the question, "What's the problem with Qi?" The next question is, "How was the problem created?" or "Where did the problem come from?"

These questions and answers lead to a diagnosis and a treatment, which I talk about in Chapter 5.

As noted in the section "Maintaining the Eight Balances," earlier in this chapter, you don't necessarily achieve balance where all relationships and interactions are equal — but you do need enough Yin Qi or Yang Qi to maintain the status quo. Figure 2-10 illustrates this equilibrium between Yin and Yang, the foundation of TCM theory.

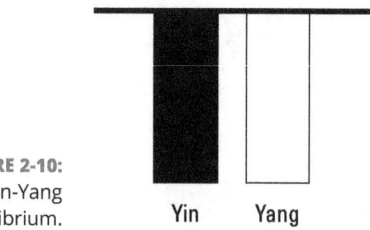

FIGURE 2-10:
Yin-Yang
equilibrium.

Yin   Yang

Not enough Qi

If the Yin Qi or Yang Qi of any organ or vital substance is insufficient, as shown in Figure 2-11, it enables one or the other to dominate or consume its counterpart. If you don't address this imbalance, the excess continues to deplete Yin or Yang Qi from one or more organ systems, and this throws off the Five Element cycle (which I talk about in the "Introducing the Five Elements" section earlier in this chapter).

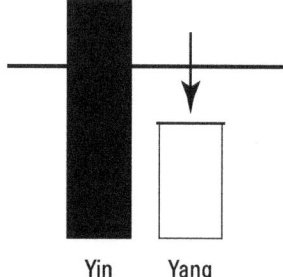

FIGURE 2-11:
Not enough Qi.

Yin   Yang

For example, insufficient Heart Yang creates excess Heart Yin that manifests as fatigue and cold limbs.

Weak Qi

A subtle difference exists between not having enough Qi (see the preceding section) and having weak Qi:

» **Not enough:** You have a shortage of supply and a high demand.

» **Weak:** Your Qi responds poorly when you need a top-notch response to fight invading pathogens.

If you have weak Yin or Yang Qi of any organ or vital substance, its counterpart can therefore exist in excess (see Figure 2-12). This relationship may not have one aggressively consuming the other, but it creates the same problem. The Yin or Yang Qi of one or more organ systems is diminished and cannot support the proper functioning of the organ system, which in turn upsets the relationships and interactions in the Five Element cycle.

Weak Heart Yin enables excess Heart Yang, which can manifest in difficulty falling asleep, while Weak Heart Yang slows blood circulation, leading to palpitations.

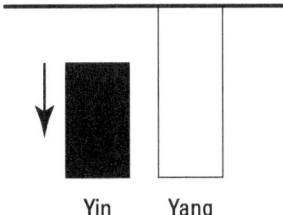

FIGURE 2-12:
Weak Qi.

Blocked Qi

When your body has a continuous and smooth flow of Qi and vital substances, it can maintain healthy function and do what it's designed to do. If this flow is fully or even partially blocked, then health issues appear. Blocked or stagnant Heart Qi hinders blood circulation, which can create chest pain or a heart attack.

Wrong-direction Qi

Healthy Qi moves in one direction. The ancient practitioners determined that the Five Elements cycle and the flow of Qi in the channels move in a specific sequence. The starting of a car engine follows a sequence of interactions. If the sequence runs out of order or backward, things can go wrong quickly.

In TCM, the Qi of each organ and vital substance has its natural direction. For example:

>> Lung Qi descends to disperse oxygen.

>> Spleen Qi ascends to distribute nutrients.

>> Small and large intestine Qi descends to eliminate waste.

As a practitioner, I have not encountered this Qi problem, but if it does happen, it can cause havoc in the cycle and lead to a variety of health problems. For example, ascending Large Intestine Qi can lead to severe constipation, and ascending Lung Qi can lead to difficulty breathing.

Chapter **3**

Accessing TCM Professionals

For any kind of personal service (health care or self-care), you probably want to do some research to find someone who's the right fit for you. For more than a decade, I've kept the same hair stylist, doctor, dentist, nail salon, car shop, dry cleaner — you get the drift — because some services shouldn't surprise you. You know you'll leave a satisfied customer.

Finding a TCM practitioner is no different. The experience and the results may be a pleasant surprise (as a patient, I have come off the table on occasion in a state of wonder at how I feel), but the ability and the knowledge of the practitioner should be something you can be confident about. Like most medical professionals, TCM practitioners are held to the same fundamental standard as any other licensed medical professionals.

The purpose of this chapter is to help you find TCM practitioners with the appropriate level of ability and judgement to assure you that your treatment and care will be safe and harmless. A little research and reaching out to one of the organizations in this chapter can help you choose the right one for you.

Looking for Licensure and Regulations

Practitioners have borrowed or adapted many of the tools and techniques in Traditional Chinese Medicine (TCM) to apply them in what I consider other delivery systems, such as physical therapy, massage, and aesthetics (for example, facials). As a TCM practitioner, I like to see these tools and techniques used to help people, and I'm committed to ensuring that only properly trained and regulated practitioners use these tools and techniques appropriately. Depending on your specific needs, you can choose the level of qualification that you want from the person delivering your TCM (or TCM-inspired) treatment.

REMEMBER

Although licensed acupuncturists receive training in all the fundamental tools and techniques of TCM, the U.S. formally regulates only acupuncture. Therefore, the discussion in the following sections mainly applies to acupuncture.

In the United States, two types of authorities regulate and license acupuncturists:

>> **At the national level:** The National Certification Commission for Acupuncture and Oriental Medicine (NCCAOM) tests and licenses practitioners in four TCM disciplines/specialties (see the section "NCCAOM Diplomate credentials," later in this chapter, for more details).

>> **At the state level:** Individual boards test and license practitioners so that they can practice in a particular state. At the time of publication, 47 states and the District of Columbia regulated acupuncture. Only Alabama, Oklahoma, and South Dakota don't have practice acts that define and regulate who can practice acupuncture and how they can practice it professionally.

REMEMBER

Practice acts are laws; they are made official with an act by the state legislature. Violations range from fines to loss of license to criminal prosecution.

TECHNICAL
STUFF

TCM practitioners in the U.S. are referred to as licensed acupuncturists with the credentials listed after their name as L.Ac. However, their education, examination, and licensing encompass a range of TCM therapies, including herbal medicine, massage (typically tui na and/or shiatsu), moxibustion, cupping, gua sha, diet and lifestyle counseling, and movement therapy such as tai chi and qi gong.

The following sections give you an overview of the NCCAOM diplomate designation, followed by a general discussion of state board licensure. Although I'm most familiar with the California Acupuncture Board (CAB) because I'm licensed in that state, I provide some general information about licensing from state boards. Achieving an NCCAOM diplomate designation represents the highest level of qualification for licensed acupuncturists in the U.S.

Understanding NCCAOM licensure

The National Certification Commission for Acupuncture and Oriental Medicine (NCCAOM) is the only organization authorized to offer national certification for acupuncture in the U.S. Established in 1982, NCCAOM develops and administers a standard examination that tests someone's competency to practice acupuncture.

AUTHOR SAYS

Essentially, passing the NCCAOM exam means that you know enough not to mess things up. That statement may sound crass or flippant, but it's the same for every licensed profession. You don't know whether your doctor passed their medical boards with flying colors or just barely squeaked by. You don't know whether your lawyer was at the top or bottom of their graduating class, but they passed the bar exam and, therefore, are duly authorized to practice law. For this reason, take a close look at a practitioner's qualifications and professional experience.

The main purpose of licensure or certification is to ensure client, consumer, and patient safety and to reduce or minimize the risk of harm. A Certified Public Accountant (CPA) has met the standard for a certain level of expertise in working with financial records and transactions. It doesn't mean that they won't miss a number or make an error on a spreadsheet, but they're less likely to make that kind of mistake. The same thinking applies to licensed acupuncturists, who have demonstrated a certain level of expertise in treating people by using needles (and other TCM tools). They might still miss an acupuncture point on your body, but their demonstrated knowledge makes that less likely to happen.

The NCCAOM also manages recertification. Most licensed or certified professionals need to maintain and expand their skills and knowledge through continuing education (CE). An NCCAOM certification is valid for four years, and licensed acupuncturists have to renew their certification before those four years elapse. They don't have to take another exam, but they do have to complete and record enough CE courses during their four-year certification period to compile the required number of CE units (CEUs). At the time I'm writing this, the NCCAOM requires a person to take 60 CEUs in those four years.

NCCAOM Diplomate Credentials

After students pass the NCCAOM exam (discussed in the preceding section), they become known as *certified Diplomates* who specialize in one of the following areas:

>> **Acupuncture:** A Diplomate of Acupuncture, or Dipl. Ac. (NCCAOM), has certification in the practice of acupuncture, which involves stimulating specific points by using needles, mild electrical stimulation (with or without needles), hand or finger pressure (acupressure), and heat (usually *moxibustion*, burning dried mugwort near points on the body). The Diplomate of Acupuncture also includes cupping and gua sha.

>> **Chinese Herbology:** A Diplomate of Chinese Herbology (also known as Chinese herbal medicine) — or Dipl. C.H. (NCCAOM) — can provide treatment by using natural materials, such as plants, roots, and minerals. You can find more details about Chinese herbal medicine in Chapter 5.

>> **Asian Bodywork Therapy:** The Diplomate of Asian Bodywork Therapy (ABT) — or Dipl. ABT (NCCAOM) — is the newest NCCAOM certification. Practitioners use ABT to treat the body, mind, and spirit through manual pressure and/or manipulation. Not all the modalities included in the Diplomate of ABT have TCM roots (for example, Traditional Thai Bodywork or Nuad Bo 'Rarn). However, they all follow TCM principles and focus on balancing energy to encourage healing. I'll share a bit on tui na (a TCM therapy) in Chapter 5.

>> **Oriental Medicine:** The Diplomate of Oriental Medicine — or Dipl. O.M. (NCCAOM) — certification indicates that the practitioner has met the standard for all three areas of TCM: acupuncture, Chinese herbology, and ABT. It's the most difficult certification to achieve and maintain because it requires the practitioner to demonstrate knowledge and competency in all three subjects, as well as biomedicine and foundational theory.

TECHNICAL STUFF

TCM students in the U.S. receive training in *acupuncture and moxibustion* and *materia medica* from accredited institutions (see "Setting the standards" later in this chapter). However, a person can become a diplomate in one or more of the subjects if desired. A separate exam is given for each of the three main subjects, with additional testing in biomedicine for the Diplomate of Oriental Medicine.

Except ABT, all the certifications require a master's degree (three to four years of academic study and hands-on or clinical practice) from an accredited TCM college or program. For national ABT certification, candidates must complete a designated number of hours of academic and practical instruction from a formal school or program. At the time of this writing, you need 500 hours of practical and theoretical instruction to qualify for certification.

Depending on the type of certification, you need to take varying levels of required coursework and clinical training in the following subjects:

>> Biomedicine (chemistry, biology, physics, and so on)

>> Anatomy and physiology

>> TCM fundamentals

   • History and theory

   • Channels and points on the body

- Herbal medicine

- Acupuncture and other techniques (including auricular (ear) acupuncture, neuroacupuncture (scalp acupuncture), cupping, and moxibustion)

» Asian Body Therapy

- Tui na

- Shiatsu

» Safety and regulations

- Herb-pharmaceutical interactions

- Clean Needle Technique (CNT; see Chapter 6)

- Red flags and referrals

» Ethics and practice management

Except for ABT, the Diplomate credentials include the abbreviation for licensed acupuncturist (L.Ac.), which is obtained from a state board that regulates TCM practice. A practitioner who has a Diplomate of Oriental Medicine would present their credentials as follows:

[*Practitioner's name*], Dipl. O.M. (NCCAOM), L.Ac.

If the practitioner has an online presence, you can look for a digital badge indicating which certification they have. They might have more than one badge, indicating multiple certifications. You can see these badges, or service marks, on the NCCAOM website (`https://www.nccaom.org/find-a-practitioner-directory`). See Figure 3-1.

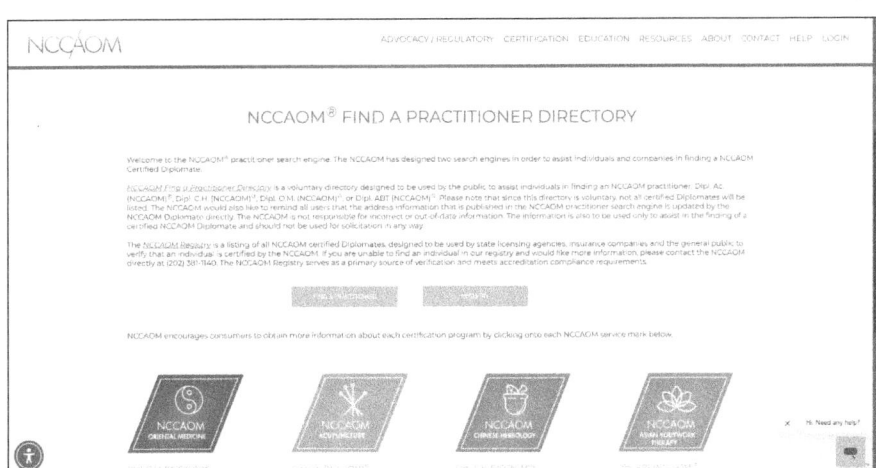

FIGURE 3-1:
The NCCAOM
website.

The NCCAOM Advantage

A TCM practitioner doesn't need an NCCAOM certification to practice in the state of their choice. They can obtain licensure by following the application process of their state's regulatory board. The conundrum here is that each state has its own regulations and requirements for acupuncture licensing and practice.

You can imagine that any process that involves an examination on a statewide basis requires a considerable amount of time and money for both the regulatory board and the applicant.

For example, a state board has to pay staff to:

>> Create the exam questions.

>> Manage and monitor applicants during the testing process.

>> Arrange for and set up an online test program and/or a room for in-person examinations.

>> Grade the exams and notify applicants of the results.

   These days, grading is done electronically, but the responses still need to be confirmed if there is uncertainty about which bubble is filled or if bubbles are not filled in properly.

>> Prepare and mail license documentation.

>> Oversee ongoing certification renewals.

The applicant's investment includes:

>> Fees for the application and exam.

>> The time it takes to study and prepare for the exam.

>> Costs for travel and accommodation if they have to take the exam in person and it isn't offered near their residence.

>> Loss of work time associated with study and examination.

>> The time, effort, and costs associated with obtaining the degree(s) that qualify them for licensure. (My student loans are no joke.)

The advantage of getting NCCAOM Diplomate status is *reciprocity* (when licensing boards accept the credentials of another licensing authority). For TCM, 47 states and the District of Columbia recognize the NCCAOM certification if someone wants to apply for a license to practice in that state or district. Although each state has different regulations, if a practitioner achieves NCCAOM certification, they don't need to take another comprehensive test. However, some states may require certified Diplomates to take a supplementary exam covering specific safety or health regulations, as well as additional requirements, to obtain a license.

For both the state board and the applicant, reciprocity cuts down on time and resources, creating a win-win process. And if practitioners want or need to move to another state, they can do so with less hassle than having to go through another state board process again.

For potential patients, finding a practitioner who has an NCCAOM certification provides the assurance that the practitioner has met the highest bar in the country for academic instruction, clinical experience, and safety and patient-care standards.

State licensing boards

The state licensing boards do what NCCAOM does, just at the state, not national, level. Forty-seven states and the District of Columbia regulate acupuncture practice. However, California is the only state that doesn't accept NCCAOM certification, which means that the state requires applicants to pass the California Acupuncture Licensing Exam (CALE), even if they already have NCCAOM certification.

The primary concern of state licensing boards is consumer safety. So, most acupuncture boards are within departments that grant licensing for many different professions. All states' acupuncture boards have common elements to their purpose and structure, which include:

>> Establishing, updating, and maintaining standards of qualification and conduct.

>> Investigating allegations of unprofessional conduct or risky/incompetent practice.

>> Taking disciplinary action against licensees who violate the regulations or code of conduct.

>> Managing the licensing and renewal process.

>> Developing and administering any examinations or testing.

>> Reviewing, evaluating, and approving training programs and continuing education unit (CEU) providers and courses.

>> Defining the scope of practice for an acupuncturist.

California defines acupuncture as a *primary health-care profession,* which means you can see an acupuncturist without having a prior diagnosis or referral by a licensed physician.

>> Determining what techniques are included in the scope of practice.

>> Comprising acupuncturists and members of the public, as appointed by the state's governor and/or legislative branches.

TCM involves more than just acupuncture, and most regulations acknowledge it to include all or some of the following:

>> Cupping

>> Moxibustion

>> Electroacupuncture

>> Asian Body Therapy (ABT)

>> Lifestyle consultation (diet, nutrition, exercise)

>> Acupressure

>> Herbs and plant/animal/mineral products of natural origin

>> Dietary supplements

TIP

If you're curious about the specific TCM regulations in your state, go to NCCAOM's interactive map. www.nccaom.org/state-licensure. Click your state to go directly to the information.

Setting the standards

To become a licensed acupuncturist, you must graduate from an accredited TCM college with a minimum of a master's degree. For educational institutions at any level, obtaining accreditation means the institution meets established standards of quality from an independent, third-party organization. Maintaining accreditation is critical to the survival of an educational institution because with accreditation comes money (and the ability of a student or their family to borrow it for study). But that's a rabbit hole for someone else to follow.

Getting the stamp of approval from the Council of Colleges of Acupuncture and Herbal Medicine

The history of accreditation for TCM programs (offered as a degree in a larger institution like Bastyr University's Acupuncture and East Asian Medicine programs) and colleges (dedicated solely to TCM) is short compared to that of traditional higher education. It began with the founding of the National Council of Acupuncture Schools and Colleges to promote educational excellence in the field.

Subsequently, it was incorporated and renamed the Council of Colleges of Acupuncture and Herbal Medicine (CCAHM). For the Western medical community to take TCM seriously and trust it as a profession, the original members of CCAHM knew that TCM education must have quality standards on par with those of traditional higher education.

To set these standards, the CCAHM established a separate accreditation commission (then known as the Accreditation Commission for Acupuncture & Oriental Medicine [ACAOM]) to develop criteria for TCM colleges and programs that applied for approval from the U.S. Department of Education. After much hard work, the CCAHM achieved its goal in 1990, when the Department of Education, as well as the Council on Post-Secondary Accreditation (a nongovernmental agency that existed from 1974 to 1993 to review and coordinate the work of accrediting agencies), recognized accreditation for acupuncture programs at the master's degree level.

In addition to serving as the standard bearer for the profession, the CCAHM maintains and administers the Clean Needle Technique (CNT) certification program, which a practitioner has to complete for licensure. For more on this specific requirement, see Chapter 6.

Since 1990, the CCAHM and its member colleges have continued to review and refine the core curriculum and expand accreditation to the doctorate level. By doing so, the CCAHM:

>> Maintains the integrity of the profession

>> Assures the continued evolution of current and future practitioners

>> Promotes greater confidence among practitioners and patients

>> Supports better access to TCM across the country

Accrediting through the ACAHM

The third-party organization overseeing TCM accreditation is the Accreditation Commission for Acupuncture and Herbal Medicine (ACAHM). As its website describes, the Department of Education recognizes the ACAHM "to serve as the nationally recognized accrediting agency of programs in acupuncture and East Asian Medicine (EAM) and institutions exclusively providing EAM-related programs."

ACAHM reviews and evaluates every aspect of the institution or program, from facilities to curriculum to faculty and staff compensation to enrollment to operating budget, and so on.

For first-timers, getting pre-accredited requires its own multistep process. An institution/program can qualify as pre-accredited for three years before moving on to the actual accreditation process. After ACAHM approves an organization, it receives accreditation for five years (seven, under certain circumstances), and then the same process starts all over again.

ACAHM is the sole accrediting agency for standalone TCM colleges such as Emperor's College in Santa Monica, California, and the New York College of Traditional Chinese Medicine in Mineola, New York. However, if an institution offers degrees in multiple fields, ACAHM can accredit only the TCM program that's part of a larger institution, such as Bastyr University's Acupuncture and East Asian Medicine Programs. For more details, you can visit ACAHM's Accreditation Procedures web page. www.acahm.org/policies/accreditation-procedures.

Promoting the profession

Despite being a trusted health-care system in other parts of the world for thousands of years, the U.S. doesn't classify acupuncture and other TCM techniques as mainstream medical treatments. Some suspect it (it's from China!). Some fear it (it's needles!). Some doubt it (it's not scientific!). Some dismiss it (there's no such thing as Qi!).

In addition to the organizations discussed throughout the section "Looking for Licensure and Regulations," earlier in this chapter, various other organizations in the U.S. work to encourage people to take a stab at TCM. For brevity's sake, I'd like to focus on two organizations that do incredible work and get the word out.

American Society of Acupuncturists

The American Society of Acupuncturists (ASA), formed in 2015, is a consortium of 37 state associations that, in total, represent over 5,000 members. (Not all states have an association, and not all state associations are ASA members.) Its continuing mission: to advocate for increased access to TCM for more people; to advance acupuncturists as valuable contributors to and partners in health care; and to boldly work to achieve *whole-person medical care* (meaning physical, mental, emotional, and spiritual) in the American health-care system.

The professional acupuncture associations in each state play a significant role in increasing public awareness, supporting practitioners by offering education and advocacy, and keeping practitioners connected and informed about important issues such as the scope of practice, state and national policy changes, new research, and challenges facing the profession. If you want to find out if your state has an ASA-affiliated association, please check the ASA website's Member State Associations page. www.asacu.org/about-us/state-organizations.

MEDICARE COVERAGE

The ASA wants to improve access to acupuncture for Medicare beneficiaries through legislative channels (meaning through Congress). Although Medicare does cover acupuncture, it doesn't recognize acupuncturists as Medicare providers. Patients have to go through a third-party, such as a hospital or other authorized provider, which creates high demand and limited appointment availability. As a result, accessing acupuncture services through the current Medicare model is far from streamlined, but at least some states' regulations allow direct access to acupuncturists.

Co-sponsored by U.S. Representatives Judy Chu (Democrat-California) and Brian Fitzpatrick (Republican-Pennsylvania), the Acupuncture for Seniors Act (House Resolution 3133), introduced by Representative Chu in May 2023 and, at the time of writing, referred to the Subcommittee on Health, would allow the Centers for Medicare and Medicaid Services (CMS) to recognize acupuncturists as Medicare providers. CMS can then provide 60 million beneficiaries with direct access to acupuncture services from those who are best qualified to provide those services.

www.asacu.org.

Society for Acupuncture Research

Founded in 1933 by an informal group of like-minded TCM practitioners and scientists, the Society for Acupuncture Research (SAR) is dedicated to evaluating and improving research for acupuncture and other TCM therapies. SAR includes institutional and individual members that represent both Eastern and Western practitioners and scientists from around the world, such as the French College of Acupuncture (https://acupuncture-medic.fr/cfa-mtc/) and the University of California, San Francisco's Osher Center for Integrative Health (http://osher.ucsf.edu).

SAR publishes the *Journal of Integrative and Complementary Medicine*, as well as a series of evidence-based assessments (evaluations of a topic or subject supported by research) that discuss acupuncture and TCM for specific conditions. SAR also organizes and sponsors international conferences that bring licensed practitioners, medical doctors, and research scientists from Eastern and Western medicine together to share and expand their knowledge to promote integrated health care for the benefit of all. www.acupunctureresearch.org.

Choosing a Licensed Acupuncturist

When you decide to see a licensed acupuncturist, you can easily find one by conducting an online search. However, choosing the first provider you see online doesn't really help you determine which provider fits your needs. First, you have to know what to look for among the candidates.

The section "Looking for Licensure and Regulations," earlier in this chapter, gives you a little information about the educational requirements for those who can treat you with acupuncture. Use that information to find a qualified practitioner. Table 3-1 provides a comparison of the level of training and education required for providers so that you can make an informed choice for yourself or a loved one.

AUTHOR SAYS

The training and education requirements in Table 3-1 are general in nature and don't encompass individual state regulations, accrediting authorities, and so on. The practitioner's education may be limited to just acupuncture or may include varying degrees of instruction in TCM theory, adjunct therapies, and diagnostics. (I go over these variations for licensed acupuncturists in the section "Looking for Licensure and Regulations," earlier in this chapter.)

TABLE 3-1   ## Training Requirements for Acupuncture Providers

Instructional Hours	Provider	Conditions Treated
3–4 years; 1,950–2,600 classroom and clinic hours, including a minimum of 450 hours in biomedical science	Licensed acupuncturist with an accredited degree and certification through national and/or state examination	A broad range of health issues, including chronic disease, pain, internal medicine, rehabilitation, and prevention
200–300 hours of acupuncture	Medical doctor, osteopath, naturopath, chiropractor	Pain, other health conditions, per the provider's area of practice and level of TCM training
50–100 hours of acupuncture	Acupuncture technician (usually in a detox or substance abuse clinic/program*) or chiropractor	Pain, addiction
40–50 hours of dry needling**	All the providers listed in the preceding rows, as well as a physical therapist and an athletic trainer	Musculoskeletal pain

*Acupuncture technicians in these clinics/programs primarily perform auricular (ear) acupuncture and are limited to stimulating five points on the ear.

**Dry needling began as the insertion of hypodermic needles into certain parts of the body without the injection of a fluid. Eventually, the hollow hypodermic needles were replaced with solid, thin acupuncture needles.

TECHNICAL STUFF

As shown in Table 3-1, other health-care providers can provide acupuncture or dry needling. The training and testing requirements for these other providers vary by state and profession, so it's best to consult your state regulations to get specific information. Some professional organizations provide this information, including:

>> The American Academy of Medical Acupuncture provides acupuncture requirements for physicians by state. `https://medicalacupuncture.org/for-physicians/acupuncture-requirements-by-state/`.

>> The American Physical Therapy Association provides dry needling regulations for physical therapists by state. `https://www.apta.org/patient-care/interventions/dry-needling/laws-by-state`.

>> The Board of Certification for the Athletic Trainer provides dry needling regulations for athletic trainers in applicable states. `https://bocatc.org/newsroom/dry-needling-state-regulation-updates/`.

The World Health Organization (WHO) recommends that medical doctors have a minimum of 200 training hours to use acupuncture as a clinical therapy. Other health professionals should receive training according to the specific application of the technique. WHO also recommends a full course of physician training of 1,500 hours.

TIP

Consider compiling a list of the qualifications that you want for your acupuncture provider before you begin your search. You may not find information on all the qualifications online, but you can certainly ask about the practitioner's qualifications in an email or on the phone.

The following sections discuss the most common places a licensed acupuncturist works. This is changing as I write this because complementary and integrative health (CIH) approaches are catching on, as noted in Chapter 1. Basically, CIH refers to those health-care systems, therapies, and techniques that are other than or outside of Western medicine.

Private practice

Most licensed acupuncturists work in private practice. Some practice solo and wear all the hats. Others form a shared practice with other licensed acupuncturists, while others may join forces with an associated professional, such as a chiropractor or massage therapist.

The National Certification Commission for Acupuncture and Oriental Medicine (NCCAOM) and the American Society of Acupuncturists (ASA) have directories of licensed acupuncturists that you can search:

>> **NCCAOM:** www.nccaom.org/find-a-practitioner-directory

>> **ASA:** www.asacu.org/find-a-practitioner

If you have a TCM college nearby, they likely have a directory of practicing alumni.

Of course, a standard online search will direct you to local practitioners. Whether you rely on reviews or not, they may be helpful in identifying a shortlist of candidates that you can cross-check on the directories above.

Community acupuncture

Community acupuncture clinics are exactly what they sound like: They offer acupuncture treatment in a communal setting, where multiple patients sit or recline in a large room to receive treatment. Community acupuncture clinics have their benefits:

>> Cost less than private sessions with an acupuncturist because a few practitioners can see several patients at a time.

>> Fees are usually based on a sliding scale or a donation.

The trade-offs are:

>> Lack of privacy

>> Abbreviated or no diagnostic examination or inquiry

>> Limited number of acupuncture point locations used

But community acupuncture can be just as effective as private treatment for a number of conditions, such as pain, addiction, and sleep or digestive issues.

The People's Organization of Community Acupuncture (POCA), a nonprofit organization dedicated to increasing affordable access to acupuncture, has a clinic finder on its website at www.pocacoop.com/places. Since 2006, POCA has provided education, training, and support for its members in best practices in creating and running a community acupuncture clinic, as well as in treatment techniques and methods. POCA-affiliated clinics adhere to the same values and standards of care as POCA itself.

Veterans Health Administration

The U.S. Department of Veterans Affairs (VA) is responsible for managing the entire system of benefits for American veterans, from housing and education to disability and health-care. The VA provides health care through the largest integrated health-care system in the U.S., the Veterans Health Administration (VHA), which operates over 1,300 facilities serving approximately 9.1 million veterans. In 2011, the VHA created its Office of Patient-Centered Care and Cultural Transformation to implement a Whole Health approach toward health care and well-being for veterans and their families.

Acupuncture became one of the complementary and integrative health (CIH) techniques in its Whole Health system in 2017, and the Under Secretary of Health of the VHA granted approval to hire licensed acupuncturists at VHA medical centers in 2018. Given the size of the VHA system, its integration of acupuncture and licensed practitioners can influence how other health-care providers and/or systems can apply, study, and expand acupuncture (and other TCM therapies) throughout the U.S. health-care system.

You can find out more about the Whole Health program at `www.va.gov/wholehealth`.

Hospital systems

More and more hospitals are taking a similar approach as the VHA (discussed in the preceding section) by placing an emphasis on more individualized, patient-focused care and the inclusion of complementary and integrative health (CIH) techniques among their services. Some hospital systems have a full CIH program (for example, University Hospitals in Cleveland, Ohio). Some establish a referral network of CIH providers that are approved for patient care (such as Kaiser Permanente in various cities). You can check your nearby hospital system's website and search for "acupuncture" to see whether they offer acupuncture treatments.

Other self-care businesses

You may be able to access acupuncture and/or other TCM and complementary and integrative health (CIH) therapies in businesses that offer other self-care services, such as:

>> Spas
>> Reflexology (foot massage) and other massage businesses

>> Gyms and health clubs

>> Nail and beauty salons

Asking about Insurance Coverage

Officially, acupuncture is the only TCM technique covered by insurance in the U.S. at the time I'm writing this book. A study published by the *Journal of the American Medical Association (JAMA)* in 2022 examined trends in insurance coverage for acupuncture from 2010 to 2019. It found coverage to be inconsistent and limited to a few specific conditions, and insurers required patients to share more of the cost than other non-drug treatments, such as chiropractic care and transcutaneous electrical nerve stimulation.

Uncovering what's covered

At the time of writing, more insurance companies are providing more coverage for acupuncture. In 2020, Medicare Part B started reimbursing patients who pay for acupuncture to treat their low back pain.

The *opioid crisis* (sudden and rapid rise of opioid addiction, overdose, and death), which the Secretary of the Department of Health and Human Services declared a public health emergency in 2017, led to efforts to find pain management alternatives. Soon after, guidelines issued by multiple federal agencies and national organizations — such as the U.S. Department of Health and Human Services, the U.S. Food and Drug Administration, The Joint Commission, the American College of Physicians, and the American Academy of Family Physicians — recommended acupuncture as part of comprehensive pain care.

With a vote of confidence from these influential organizations, it didn't take long for insurers to get with the program. But you need to do a bit of detective work to find out whether your insurance plan covers acupuncture and how much it covers. Use these resources to find the answers:

>> **Review your insurance provider's documentation.** Start with the benefits summary to see whether it includes acupuncture. If it doesn't, don't despair. The benefits summary typically includes the most requested benefits. Find your evidence of coverage (EOC) document (or request one). The EOC provides a complete description of your coverage, co-payments, exclusions, and limitations.

>> **Visit your insurance company's website.** Log in to your account to find your plan's acupuncture benefits, including your co-pay, your allotted number of visits, and whether your plan covers out-of-network providers. Search for in-network acupuncturists (and out-of-network ones, as needed).

Alternatively, you can call your insurance company's customer service department if you need help accessing this information.

>> **Ask your primary care doctor whether they can recommend any acupuncture providers.** Some may have personal experience themselves, or one of their staff members or other patients may know of someone. Some won't know anything about acupuncture. Some will be skeptical and may suggest another option. You never know what their response will be until you ask. You're the decision-maker, so you decide if their response is acceptable or if you want to seek a second opinion.

>> **Ask your HR department or a co-worker.** They may have personal experience with a provider already on your plan, or they may have already gone through a process to find one.

>> **Contact acupuncture providers in your area and verify whether they take your insurance plan.** If acupuncture isn't covered in your plan, see "Advocating for Coverage" next.

TIP

If you don't have insurance, you can ask whether the provider has a lower fee option. We can't discount our fees, but we can charge less if warranted. I can't speak for all providers, but in my practice, I offer a new patient package in which I charge less than what is customary and usual for three follow-up visits after the initial visit. I also offer a financial hardship agreement that sets an affordable rate for a set period of time (for example, three months) or a set number of treatments (for example, four).

Acupuncture is an eligible medical expense for Flexible Spending Accounts (FSAs), Health Savings Accounts (HSAs), and Health Reimbursement Arrangements (HRAs). You may need a Letter of Medical Necessity (LMN) from your doctor to show that you need acupuncture for a specific medical condition. The LMN is like a prescription and should include the need for acupuncture treatment, the frequency of treatment, and how long you need to receive it. For example:

"Jane Doe has acute back pain and doesn't react well to pain medicine, so acupuncture is a viable alternative for her. She should receive weekly treatment until her pain is well controlled."

WARNING

Acupuncture is not eligible for reimbursement with a Limited-Purpose Flexible Spending Account (LPFSA) or a Dependent Care Flexible Spending Account (DCFSA).

Advocating for coverage

If your insurance provider doesn't currently provide coverage for acupuncture, you can:

>> **Request coverage.** Ask the insurance provider to consider covering acupuncture by writing a letter or email to your plan administrator. If you have insurance through your employer, you can ask your employer to inquire, too.

>> **Create a petition.** Others who have your insurance plan may also want coverage that includes acupuncture, so a petition for coverage may help get everyone on the plan covered.

>> **Contact your state acupuncture association.** They can probably give you pointers on how to advocate for coverage.

2

Exploring TCM Treatments

IN THIS PART . . .

Understand the what, where, when, how, and why of acupuncture and the way it affects your body

Explore the range of TCM treatments available to you from a licensed practitioner

Become familiar with the TCM treatment process and how to prepare for your treatment experience

Chapter **4**

Understanding Acupuncture

Acupuncture is a healing art that involves the stimulation of specific points on the body. Practitioners can produce the stimulation by using needles, heat, manual pressure, electric current, or other means, but most acupuncturists stimulate by needling. This stimulation can help normalize body functions, reduce pain, and treat certain diseases or bodily dysfunctions.

No one can pinpoint when and where people began to use acupuncture. Some research articles and TCM history texts refer to notes written on turtle shells that indicate humans have used acupuncture for over 4,000 years, but the consensus estimate is around 3,000 years, give or take a few hundred years. Also, no one has a definitive answer about the necessity that mothered the invention of acupuncture, other than the age-old human quest to fix what's broken.

Because acupuncture is the best-known TCM therapy and most used in the U.S., I cover it in this chapter as comprehensively as I can. I discuss the other therapies in Chapter 5.

Getting Blood with a Stone: Ancient Origins

TCM scholars and researchers who wrote the TCM textbooks used in the U.S. today know that acupuncture evolved from bloodletting with stone instruments, which was used in many ancient cultures, based on historical records. Archaeologists discovered *bian* stone needles (named for the type of stone used) of 2 to 3½ inches in Neolithic (10,000–2,200 BCE) ruins and graves in China. Several of these needles were found in Inner Mongolia and Shandong Province. At one end, they had a semicircular edge or three edges; the other end was pyramid- or cone-shaped. Ancient medical texts describe people using the pyramid- or cone-shaped ends for bloodletting and the edged ends to open and drain boils or abscesses.

While humanity developed new materials and manufacturing techniques, the needles got thinner (phew!) and came in a variety of metals, such as bronze, silver, and gold. Chinese doctors began keeping medical records sometime in the 5th century BCE, according to ancient documents. Excavated from a Han Dynasty tomb in Hunan Province, two silk scrolls written in the 3rd century BCE offer the earliest known documentation of *meridians* and *collaterals* (main channels or pathways for the circulation of Qi and Blood) — see Chapter 2 — and smaller branches or supplemental pathways for the circulation of Qi and Blood.

The Holy Grail of TCM diagnosis and treatment is a two-part book known to every TCM practitioner as the *Huang Di Nei Jing* (or simply *Nei Jing*), which translates to *The Yellow Emperor's Inner Canon*. As legend goes, Emperor Huangdi, who reigned in China from 2697 to 2597 BCE, wrote this text as a reflection on health and disease. In a way, it's like another emperor's classic — *Meditations* by Roman emperor Marcus Aurelius, which offers a discussion of how to live a healthy and meaningful life. Figure 4-1 shows a later dynastic copy of the *Huang Di Nei Jing*.

The two parts of the *Nei Jing* include:

>> *Basic Questions (Su Wen):* Written as a dialogue between Huangdi and his physician, the Basic Questions text provides the philosophical side of TCM — addressing the principles of health, disease, and treatment; presenting the underlying theories of Yin-Yang, the Five Elements, and Qi (check out Chapter 2 for discussion of these TCM concepts); exploring contributing disease factors, such as external pathogens, emotions, lifestyle, and diet; and reviewing the organ and meridian systems.

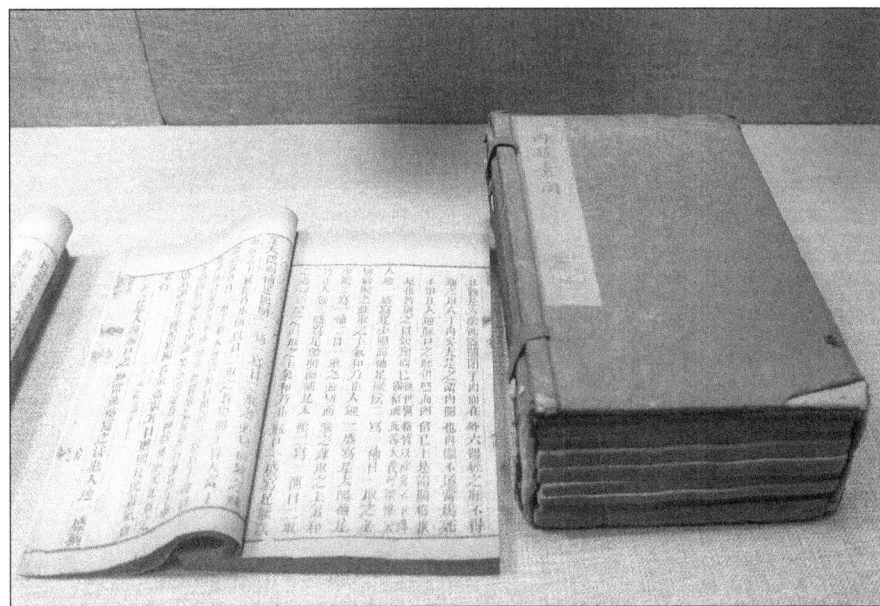

FIGURE 4-1:
A later dynastic copy of the *Huang Di Nei Jing.*

>> *Spiritual Pivot (Ling Shu)*: The Spiritual Pivot text deals with the practical side of TCM — focusing on acupuncture and *moxibustion* (burning dried mugwort near points on the body) to treat various diseases. It details the meridian system and Qi flow, and it offers guidance on needle technique and point selection.

Despite being attributed to Emperor Huangdi, the book is likely the work of several authors. Regardless, it remains the foundation of TCM theory and application to this day.

Bringing Acupuncture (and TCM) Westward

Physicians over millennia considered, reconsidered, and refined the classic text *Huang Di Nei Jing* (which you can read about in the preceding section), adding to and expanding the library of TCM resources and references. The Chinese medicine formulated and practiced in the 17th century made its way westward through European trade and missionaries. Dutch physician Willem ten Rhijne wrote the first Western discussion of acupuncture in the 1670s, titled *De acupunctura* (*The acupuncture*). Rhijne studied Chinese medicine for two years while he worked for the East India Company in Nagasaki, Japan.

Supposedly, the English brought more than tea and taxes to the American colonies, but Chinese medicine was more of a curiosity than a healing system. Fast forward a century or so, when Chinese emigrants flocked to California, which they described as the Gold Mountain, to escape famine and political unrest, and to seek their fortune in gold mines or to earn money working on farms and along railroad tracks. In addition to their dreams of a better life, they brought the healing arts of their homeland. Initially, they used their Chinese medicine to treat themselves. Over time and assimilation, practitioners used their Chinese medicine to treat non-Chinese people, and a new version (for lack of a better word) of Chinese medicine began to emerge in the U.S.

As noted earlier in this section, the material for acupuncture needles evolved from stone to metal. Early needles were made of a single metal, like bronze or gold (for royalty). Later, needles were made of steel with handles made of other metals, like copper. Today, needles are made of stainless steel and individually packaged like the ones shown in Figure 4-2.

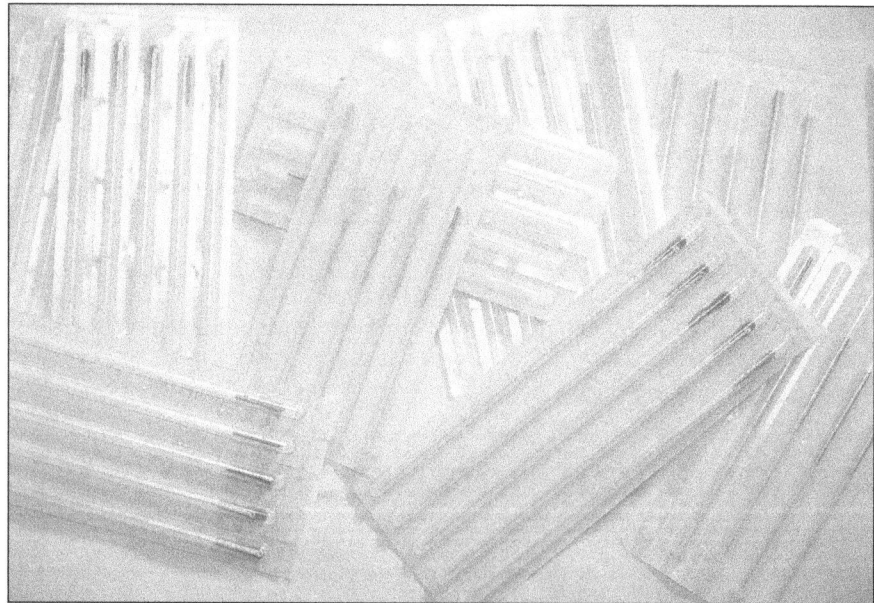

FIGURE 4-2: Stainless steel needles color-coded to indicate length and thickness.

ManuPadilla/Adobe Stock Photos

A presidential connection

From 1949 onward, Chinese medicine in China had a revolution of its own under Communist rule (a topic that someone else can tackle). When President Richard Nixon went to China in 1971 to renew Sino-American relations, a number of Americans became familiar with TCM during the trip:

>> **James Reston:** A *New York Times* reporter who experienced TCM firsthand and wrote an article about it. Reston suffered acute *appendicitis* (an inflamed appendix) and needed emergency surgery. In his article, Reston described how acupuncture and moxibustion helped alleviate his postoperative pain and discomfort.

>> **Dr. W. Kenneth Riland:** After observing Chinese medical practices during the visit, Riland, one of Nixon's doctors on the trip, stated in an interview that "acupuncture is going to be one of the greatest contributions that any group of people has made to the future of all medicine, if it is handled correctly by the people of the Western world."

>> **Major General Walter R. Tkach:** Another of Nixon's doctors who wrote the article "I Watched Acupuncture Work" in the July 1972 issue of *Reader's Digest,* further fueling interest from the medical community, as well as the general public.

First U.S. clinic and new regulations

As a result of public interest, the first major acupuncture clinic opened in New York City in July 1972, founded by three medical doctors: Yao Wu Lee, Arnold Benson, and Charles Newmark. The clinic relocated to Washington, D.C., in December 1972.

The Washington Acupuncture Center clinic soon had plenty of patients and press, treated up to 1,000 patients a day from all over the country, and employed up to 65 practitioners and staff. The Center's success was short-lived because it faced challenges from the medical board in D.C. and closed in 1974. Despite this setback, TCM in the U.S. took a small step forward when the U.S. Immigration Board added acupuncturists to its list of recognized occupations in 1973.

The story behind the first state to regulate and recognize acupuncture as a medical treatment has a plot worthy of a Korean television drama. An attorney (Arthur Steinberg), a Chinese medicine doctor (Dr. Lok Yee-Kung), and a lobbyist (James Joyce — no relation to the Irish author) wanted to set a precedent by introducing legislation in Nevada to legalize acupuncture performed by licensed acupuncturists and remove the restriction of acupuncture as a practice only medical doctors could perform.

Steinberg and Joyce arranged to have Dr. Lok demonstrate acupuncture across the street from the Nevada State Legislature before the acupuncture bill was due for a vote. Lok picked 70 volunteers from among a crowd of over 1,000 people; 30 of them just happened to be legislators. The first law that allowed non-medical doctors to practice acupuncture legally received only two nay votes in the Nevada State Senate and House combined. In subsequent years, other states quickly followed; most recently, Wyoming in 2017. All in all, 47 states and the District of Columbia have acupuncture laws on the books at the time I'm writing.

Despite its growing acceptance, interest in the formal medical community waxed and waned because of a lack of evidence-based research (that is, trials and studies that provide numbers and percentages that prove that acupuncture does work). I talk more about research in the section "Understanding what the research says," later in this chapter.

Still illegal but highly effective

I believe it was the power of the people — both practitioners and patients — that kept acupuncture and TCM alive to eventually thrive in the U.S. One such practitioner was Dr. Miriam Lee (1926–2009), whose clinic was in Palo Alto, California. Lee was a nurse, midwife, and acupuncturist in Asia before immigrating to the U.S. in 1969. Unfortunately, she couldn't use her skills while living in America because the medicine she practiced was illegal. Instead, she worked on an assembly line for Hewlett-Packard. But as a healer by trade and nature, she noticed how neighbors, friends, and co-workers suffered from ailments that she knew she could help them with.

Even though her practicing broke the law, Lee saw as many as 75 to 80 people a day, seven days a week, in her home. An ally came to her aid in the form of a local doctor, Dr. Harry Oxenhandler, who offered his office to her during his off-hours. But the powers that be didn't appreciate Lee's work. She was arrested in 1974 for practicing medicine without a license and released on bail; she faced six months in jail if convicted at her hearing. For his kindness, Oxenhandler's license was suspended. Her hearing was a bit of a sensation because patients flooded the courtroom to protest her arrest and presented themselves as proof of her healing skills. (Even the presiding judge's wife was one such patient!)

In response to increasing public attention, days after the hearing, California Governor Ronald Reagan signed legislation that made acupuncture an "experimental procedure." With this provision, Lee was able to see patients, and Oxenhandler's license was reinstated. When the California government legalized acupuncture in 1976, Lee was among the first cohort of licensed acupuncturists. She made numerous subsequent contributions to the profession.

The first accredited acupuncture schools opened in the U.S. in the late 1970s and early 1980s, and practitioners established state and national acupuncture organizations to educate, advocate, and promulgate. (For more on this topic, please see Chapter 3.)

The Food and Drug Administration didn't classify acupuncture needles as medical devices until 1996. So, acupuncture as an official medical procedure in the U.S. is younger than Taylor Swift.

Explaining How Acupuncture Works

Medical researchers (East and West), biotechnology and pharmaceutical scientists, and TCM educators and practitioners continue to investigate numerous theories about how and why acupuncture and TCM work. For example, one theory involves *embryology* (studying the development of an embryo from ovum fertilization through to the fetal stage).

Here's my interpretation of what I've read about this theory. When the sperm fertilizes an egg, two individual entities combine to become something called a single-celled zygote, just like Yang and Yin combine to be the foundation of all things. (You can read about maintaining the eight balances in Chapter 2.) This single cell divides into two cells — which divide to become four, eight, sixteen, and so on — until it is a ball of thousands and thousands of cells. The ball attaches to the womb, and the cells start to organize into a person with a brain, a spine, limbs, internal organs, skin, and so on. Somehow, they know where to go and what to do. The impetus for this replication and organization is invisible and intangible, but it exists, or none of us would be here. This is Qi (see the discussion of the Vital Three in Chapter 2); specifically, pre-natal Qi (the Qi you inherit from your parents and ancestors). The theory goes on to discuss organs and their corresponding channels (read about the major channels in Chapter 2), and so on.

When I give my Acupuncture 101 presentation at community or corporate health fairs, I explain the theories that align with my personal understanding of the three systems that are activated by acupuncture:

>> **The nervous system:** Your brain, spinal cord, and an intricate web of nerves control all your body functions.

>> **The immune system:** Your body's defense against disease includes special cells like white blood cells, proteins like antibodies, tissues like lymph nodes, and organs like the pancreas.

>> **The fascial system:** Every part of your body is covered by thin connective tissue (like plastic wrap) known as fascia that provides stability and structure to everything from bones and organs to nerves and muscles.

You may already be familiar with the first two, but the third is a system I was ignorant of until I went to TCM school. It's a system so critical to our bodies that I was shocked I didn't know it. I go over each of these systems and how acupuncture interacts with them in the following sections.

Stimulating the nervous system

Your nervous system includes your brain, spinal cord, and nerve network (see Figure 4-3):

>> **Brain:** Like the central processing unit (CPU) of your body — telling it what, when, and how to do everything, from breathing and walking to feeling and thinking.

>> **Spinal cord:** Acts as the highway that moves messages back and forth between your brain and the network of nerves.

>> **Nerves:** This network carries messages back and forth between your spinal cord and the rest of your body.

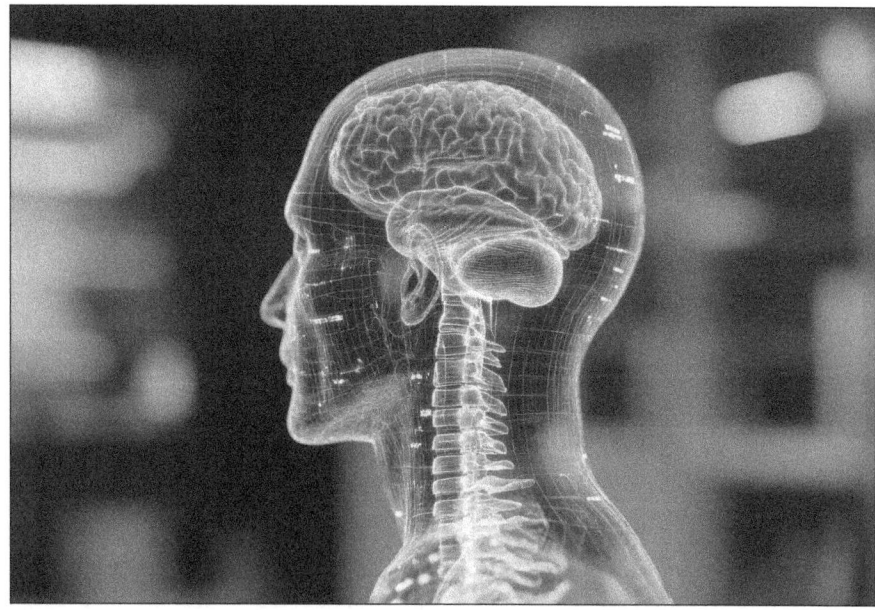

FIGURE 4-3: The nervous system transmits signals from your brain to your body through the spinal cord and its offshoots.

teera/Adobe Stock Photos

The nerve cells that make up this incredible system are called *neurons.* They transmit electrical impulses and chemical signals to and from your brain. Science has identified thousands of different neuron types, but they tend to fall into one of three categories:

>> **Sensory neurons:** Take cues from the physical and chemical inputs coming from outside your body, so you can sense what's going on around you and respond (if needed or desired). Sound, touch, and light are physical inputs, and smell and taste are chemical inputs.

>> **Motor neurons:** Help your brain and spinal cord talk to your body to enable voluntary (walking, eating) and involuntary (breathing, heart beating) movements.

>> **Interneurons:** The most common type of neuron. They connect the sensory and motor neurons. For example, if you hear (sensory) a fire alarm and smell (sensory) smoke, you get up (motor) immediately and get out (motor). If your interneurons don't relay the messages, you're toast.

Acupuncture intercepts and modifies the messages sent through this complex circuitry. I suspect that acupuncture works by influencing the interneurons because a 2024 review published in *Frontiers in Neurology* indicated that acupuncture activates "neuronal pathways" that transmit and receive signals related to pain, emotion, cognition, and the reward system that regulates pleasure.

If you've played a game of telephone, you know how mixed up the original message can get after it passes through the brains and lips of multiple people. If you play telephone while wearing earplugs, imagine how the message might get really misinterpreted. This confusion can be hilarious when you're playing a game. But if your brain and your body aren't getting the right messages, you have a serious problem!

So, acupuncture helps clear up garbled messages, or it bridges any gaps in the connections. Sometimes, acupuncture says, "Hey, lungs, inhale more deeply." Or "Hey, kidney, did you get bladder's message about slowing your roll?" Or "Hey, sensory neurons, turn down the volume on knee pain."

TECHNICAL STUFF

In an Acupuncture Now Foundation *white paper* (an in-depth, research-based report) titled "Acupuncture: More than Pain Management," by Matthew Bauer, L.Ac. (U.S.), and Mel Hopper Koppelman, M.Sc. (U.K.), they articulate this theory best: "[A]cupuncture hacks into the systems that monitor and adjust the body's own resources, thus facilitating self-healing and symptom management."

Activating the immune system

Your immune system protects you against all manner of things that can make you sick. As humans, we have three types of immunity:

>> **Natural immunity:** A type of general protection that you're born with; for example, your skin acts as a barrier against germs. Natural (or innate) immunity helps your body recognize foreign and/or potentially dangerous invaders.

>> **Adaptive immunity:** Develops throughout your life when you're exposed to disease-causing microbes, or you receive a vaccine that introduces all or parts of such microbes to your system. After your immune system gets exposure to a microbe, it adapts to recognize that particular microbe and fight it off.

>> **Passive immunity:** A borrowed form of immunity that lasts for a short time. For example, breast milk gives a baby temporary immunity to microbes that the mother's immune system can fight, allowing the baby's system to recognize and respond to those same disease-causing microbes.

This ingenious defense system seeks and destroys outside invaders (such as germs, bacteria, foreign bodies [such as splinters], and so on) by using a sophisticated army of white blood cells (WBCs), also known as leukocytes. The WBC army has two main divisions, and each division has specialty units (see Figure 4-4):

>> **Division 1:** Contains *lymphocytes,* WBCs that remember and recognize previous invaders (generally known as *antigens*):

- *The first unit: B cells* are lymphocytes that find antigens and lock onto them like the illuminated red dot from a gun, marking them for destruction. B cells keep a database of all past invaders, so if those invaders show up again, the B cells can block or target them faster.

- *The second unit:* After the B cells identify an antigen, the *T cells* mobilize to destroy it. The T-cell unit has three subgroups: helper T cells that signal other cells to neutralize invaders; cytotoxic (*cyto* meaning cell and *toxic* meaning poisonous or harmful) T cells, or "killer T cells"; and regulatory T cells (or suppressor cells) that keep the other T cells from attacking your healthy cells.

>> **Division 2:** Contains *phagocytes,* WBCs that surround and consume bacteria and other small particles (such as dust or toxins). I envision phagocyte units as a swarm of Pac-Man characters chewing up dangerous stuff while they travel through the bloodstream.

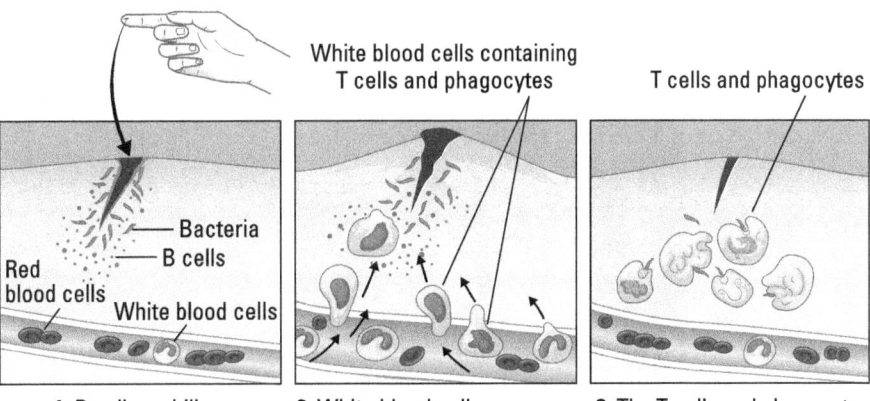

FIGURE 4-4:
WBCs rallying
to the spot
where a splinter
pricked a finger.

1. B cells mobilize.

2. White blood cells containing T cells and phagocytes join the attack. The site is swollen and inflamed from the battle.

3. The T cells and phagocytes consume the bacteria as the site heals.

When the stainless steel of an acupuncture needle pierces the barrier of your skin, your ever-alert immune system detects an invader and mobilizes its forces to seek and destroy. In my mind, acupuncture calls attention to areas that need a little reinforcement and activates the WBC army for healing and regeneration.

Facilitating through fascia

Fascia, connective tissue that surrounds and separates all components of your body, does its work and gets little notice, even though, without it, you literally can't hold yourself together. Think of your skin like an outer casing on a sausage. All the muscles, tendons, bones, veins, arteries, organs, nerve fibers, and so on, stuffed under the skin, are held in place by fascia. Fascia looks like a spider web of silly putty (see Figure 4-5). It's stringy, stretchy, slippery, smooth, and strong.

Healthy fascia allows your joints, bones, muscles, and organs to glide and slide next to each other without causing chafing, irritation, or (worse) damage. It provides stability and structure, form and function, and continuous connection for every tissue and organ in your body. When it's not healthy, fascia gets dry, rough, tight, and stiff. Think of rubber bands that lose their elasticity and snap; wet shoelaces that dry and contract so much that you can't untie them; or your own chapped lips and aching knuckles and knees.

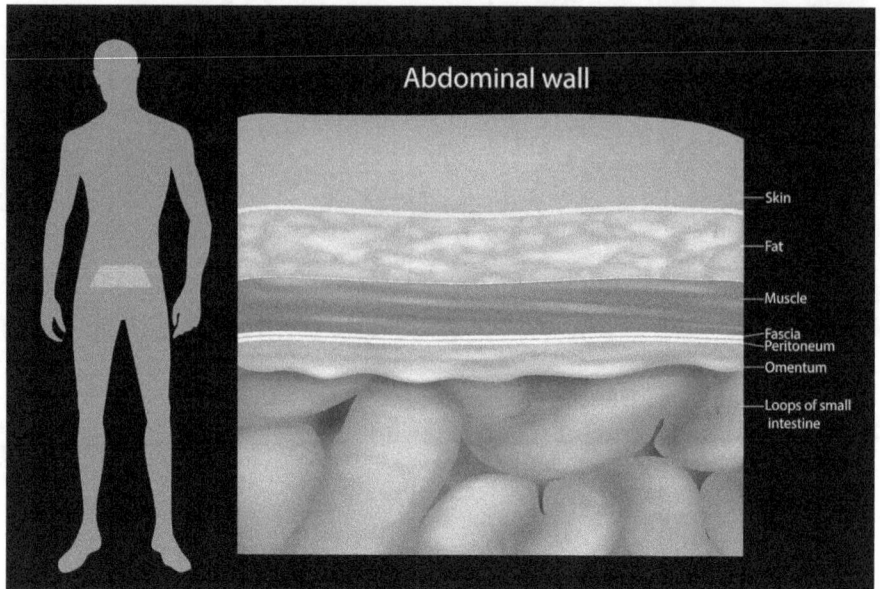

Abdominal wall

Skin
Fat
Muscle
Fascia
Peritoneum
Omentum
Loops of small
intestine

FIGURE 4-5:
Fascia that surrounds all structures, from a blood cell to an organ, looks like a web of silly putty.

sakurra/Adobe Stock Photos

Fascia contains nerves, which communicate through electrical impulses or messages sent through your nervous system (which I discuss in the section "Stimulating the nervous system," earlier in this chapter). Because fascia exists in every part of your body, it seems plausible that nerves can transmit signals through fascia. And therefore, acupuncture facilitates this communication, lining up disconnected sockets, resetting circuit breakers, pinpointing the location of damaged wires, and so on.

Understanding what the research says

When some people see (sensory neurons) the word *research,* they may immediately turn the page (motor neurons); but Western medicine and science rely on research to prove how and why things work or don't; establish standards and procedures; and validate cause-and-effect relationships. Therefore, here's a list of diseases, conditions, and symptoms that researchers have proven acupuncture (and other TCM therapies) can effectively treat and relieve:

» Adverse reactions and/or side effects to radiotherapy and/or chemotherapy, including:

- Fatigue

- Loss of appetite

- Nausea
- Neuropathy

» Allergic rhinitis (including hay fever)

» *Biliary colic* (bile duct obstruction or gallstones)

» Cardiovascular disease (stroke)

» Cognitive impairment (dementia, Alzheimer's, Parkinson's)

» Dental pain and jaw dysfunction

» Depression (including depressive neurosis and depression following stroke)

» Diabetes

» Dysentery (bacterial)

» *Dysmenorrhea* (cramping and pain during menstruation)

» Facial pain

» Headache

» Hypertension/hypotension (high/low blood pressure)

» Knee pain

» Leukopenia (reduced WBCs)

» Low back pain

» Malposition of fetus (such as breech)

» Nausea and vomiting (including morning sickness)

» Neck pain

» Osteoarthritis

» Pain in the abdomen (such as pain caused by an ulcer, or acute and chronic *gastritis* [inflammation of the stomach lining])

» *Periarthritis* (buildup of calcium crystals) in the shoulder

» Postoperative pain

» *Renal colic* (urinary tract obstruction)

» Rheumatoid arthritis

» Sciatica

» Tennis elbow

According to the World Health Organization, acupuncture and TCM have demonstrated a healing effect in another 54 diseases, conditions, and symptoms, as presented in journals and symposiums around the world. The Veterans Health Administration prepared an "Evidence Map of Acupuncture" (the Map) in 2014 as a broad overview of acupuncture and its effectiveness. The Department's researchers identified and reviewed hundreds of published research articles on acupuncture between 2005 and 2013, focusing on three areas of treatment — Pain, Wellness, and Mental Health. Although the Map showed positive evidence for acupuncture's efficacy in all three areas, the Department's researchers didn't make a definitive conclusion. They noted that scientists are continuing to research TCM and its components, but studies need better quality design and reporting.

I have notifications set for new articles on TCM and related topics on various sites such as the National Institutes of Health, DeepDyve, and the Society of Acupuncture Research. In the time I've been writing, research articles kept popping into my inbox left and right. While I'm not qualified to judge the quality of this new research, I can attest to the fact that the evidence base is growing.

TIP

Part 3 of this book provides an overview of acupuncture and TCM for several common or most worrisome diseases, conditions, and symptoms that impact people and the health-care system.

Healing with Other Types of Acupuncture

Although practitioners can perform acupuncture on any part of the body, some practitioners have dedicated themselves to studying, refining, and practicing the art of needling for specific body regions or developing other systems or styles of acupuncture. For the purposes of this book, I introduce these fully formed therapies of their own to you because you may encounter one or more of these therapies on your acupuncture journey.

Needling your ears

Ear acupuncture or *auriculotherapy,* which is stimulating specific points on the ear, is as old as acupuncture itself. Yet it wasn't until the 20th century that TCM practitioners formalized it as a distinct form of therapy. Ancient Chinese and Egyptian healers considered the ear a critical therapeutic and diagnostic tool. The *Nei Jing* (which I talk about in the section "Getting Blood with a Stone: Ancient Origins," earlier in this chapter) observed a correlation between the ear and all the organs. Later texts specified that this correlation extended to the meridians and other tissues of the body. Zhenjun Zhang, a Qing Dynasty physician, published the first auricular map of the five major organs (Lung, Spleen, Heart, Liver, and Kidney; you can read about how TCM addresses these five major organs in Chapter 2) in 1888 in his book *Essential Techniques for Massage (Lizheng anmo yaosu)*.

In 17th-century Europe, *ear cauterization* (a process of burning or dissolving tissue of the ear) was documented as a treatment for head and tooth pain, as well as for *sciatica* (irritation, inflammation, pinching, or compression of one or more nerves running down the lower back and legs). In France, local healers commonly used ear cauterization for centuries. When the formal medical community caught wind of it in the mid-1800s, some embraced and used it, while others found it alarming and warned against it. (Guess which side prevailed.) The lid was closed on the discussion and study of ear cauterization among French university circles for almost a century.

Enter Dr. Paul Nogier, a physician from Lyon, France, who also happened to study acupuncture and manual therapy like massage. In 1951, Nogier noticed a bright red scar on his patient's ear. The patient explained it was from a treatment that he received from a healer in Marseilles that cured his sciatica. A few weeks later, Nogier saw another patient sporting the same ear scar. This patient also had chronic sciatica and was relieved of it by the same Marseilles healer.

Cue montage of Nogier compiling case studies from the Marseilles healer, conducting further research, and experimenting with ear points. He meticulously mapped sensitive, responsive places on the ear that corresponded with the spinal column and body organs. In 1957, Nogier published his first ear map in a German publication, *Deutsche Zeitschrift für Akupunktur* (translated as *The German Journal of Acupuncture*).

Nogier continued to expand on his work, and other scholars and doctors in China, Europe, and the U.S. have built upon it. However, TCM researchers in China and Europe recognize Nogier for creating the foundation for ear acupuncture as a fully realized form of TCM therapy. Michael Greenwood, a noted ear researcher, expressed this clearly in an article for the *American Journal of Acupuncture*: "In a stroke, Nogier transformed ear acupuncture from an esoteric field into a simple and powerful modality" that offers the following advantages for both the practitioner and the patient:

>> You can master and administer it easily; patients can perform it at home with the proper materials and instruction. You don't need expensive tools and materials (needles, seeds, pellets, magnets, and so on).

>> You can use it as a standalone therapy or in addition to other therapies (Eastern and Western).

>> It has no negative effects (unless used improperly; for example, applying too many needles or seeds, which can lead to overstimulation, or reusing needles, which can lead to infection).

>> You can use it for a range of conditions that involve physical, emotional, and mental pain and suffering — from musculoskeletal and nerve pain to depression, addiction, and trauma, all of which you can read about in Part 3.

Present-day ear maps vary according to who developed them; for example, Nogier's successors in European schools use a map that's different from those developed in China. The ear map that I know best is from *Chinese Acupuncture and Moxibustion* (*CAM* to TCM practitioners, teachers, and students), the primary textbook from China used in the U.S. (and other countries') curriculum, and the basis of U.S. licensing examinations. The ear map shown in Figure 4-6 illustrates how acupuncture points correspond to body parts and systems.

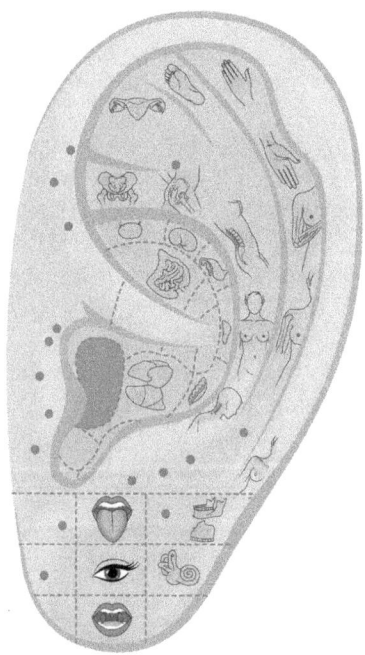

FIGURE 4-6:
Acupuncture points on the ear.

mrs_bazilio/Adobe Stock Photos

Using your head

Classic Chinese and Western medical literature include numerous references to needling the head, but *neuroacupuncture* (stimulating traditional scalp points based on neurology and neurological functions; also called *Chinese scalp acupuncture*) is the youngest therapy in the TCM toolkit. This relatively modern therapy (developed in China in the 1950s) integrates traditional Chinese needling with Western knowledge of the cerebral cortex.

TECHNICAL STUFF

The cerebral cortex is the wrinkled-looking top layer of nerve cell tissue of the brain, and this layer has four lobes (sections). Each lobe processes different information that contributes to brain function. Collectively, they control language, memory, reasoning, thought, learning, decision-making, emotion, intelligence, and personality.

Like with ear acupuncture (flip back to the preceding section for discussion of the ear), Chinese physicians started mapping areas on the scalp and which sections of the brain and body exhibited a response. The recognized founder of Chinese scalp acupuncture was neurosurgeon Dr. Jiao Shun-fa, who systematically explored and charted which specific area of the scalp aligned with which part of the brain and nervous system. He published his work in the late 1970s and presented it at the first International Acupuncture Conference held by the World Federation of Acupuncture-Moxibustion Societies (WFAS) in Beijing, China, in 1987.

Since then, the experience of scalp acupuncture specialists(often referred to as neuro-acupuncturists) and further research have improved the therapy's techniques and broadened its application. Initially used to treat post-stroke paralysis and speech loss, practitioners now use scalp acupuncture for pain management, brain and spinal cord injuries, multiple sclerosis (MS), Parkinson's disease, and mental health disorders.

Scalp acupuncture has similar advantages to ear acupuncture (easy for a practitioner to learn, inexpensive, can work as individual or combined therapy, and has minimal side effects), but with a few differences.

Although rooted in TCM, scalp acupuncture is based on the anatomy and physiology of the nervous system and not the TCM channels. (Check out Chapter 2 for more on TCM channels.) So, a neuro-acupuncturist chooses a region on the scalp according to the *cortical homunculus* (from the Latin for "outer covering" and "little man") — a visual depiction of the motor and sensory functions of the cerebral cortex. The motor and sensory nerves use different kinds of pathways in the cerebral cortex, as illustrated in Figure 4-7.

TECHNICAL STUFF

A non-specialized TCM practitioner can perform scalp acupuncture, too. However, they will choose points according to channel theory (see Chapter 2) with consideration for brain function and structure.

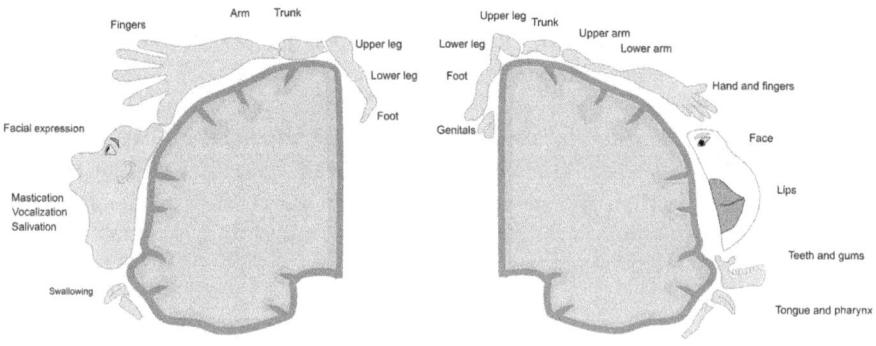

Motor areas   Sensory areas

Fingers
Arm   Trunk
Upper leg
Lower leg
Foot
Facial expression
Mastication
Vocalization
Salivation
Swallowing

Upper leg   Trunk
Lower leg   Upper arm
Foot   Lower arm
Genitals   Hand and fingers
            Face
            Lips
            Teeth and gums
            Tongue and pharynx

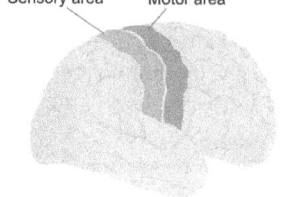

Sensory area   Motor area

FIGURE 4-7:
This motor
and sensory
homunculus
shows the areas
of the cerebral
cortex and their
corresponding
functions/organs.

ellepigrafica/Adobe Stock Photos

WARNING

Scalp acupuncture cannot and should not be practiced without an acupuncture license. Do not try this at home!

Unlike traditional acupuncture, a neuro-acupuncturist needles a motor or sensory region, instead of single points, so the practitioner can administer the therapy more easily and quickly.

**AUTHOR
SAYS**

Like ear acupuncture, neuro-acupuncture is quite portable, so the practitioner can go to the patient instead of the other way around. (As an intern, I had the privilege of treating patients in their beds with scalp acupuncture at a traumatic brain injury unit of a major San Francisco hospital.)

Revealing family secrets: Master Tung's Acupuncture

Before the ascendance of Mao Zedong to power in China in 1949, families of medical scholars taught, refined, and practiced what I consider Classical Chinese Medicine. This is the medical system documented in the *Nei Jing* (see "Getting Blood with a Stone," earlier in this chapter) and passed down through the ages by the dynastic physicians and medical scholars.

Each family closely guarded their skills and wisdom, sharing them only through the family's line of descendants. In addition, these practitioners primarily treated rich city folks. Mao's Cultural Revolution targeted what it called this elite exclusivity, and the government made every attempt to destroy it — closing Chinese medicine schools; burning ancient medical texts; persecuting (and even killing) elderly masters; and sending urban practitioners to rural areas throughout China to treat lower-income people.

Master Tung's Acupuncture, a system created by Tung Ching-Chang, originated from medical knowledge passed exclusively through generations of the Tung family. This knowledge was shared in oral verses like a recited poem. Born in 1916, Tung Ching-Chang began practicing his family's medical verses at the young age of 18, and he treated patients regardless of their ability to pay. While Mao's policies fractured Classical Chinese Medicine (among other things), Tung moved to Taiwan, where he spent the rest of his life treating patients from all classes, as well as teaching his medicine to others.

Through his clinical experience, Master Tung refined and expanded on his family's healing art to create a style of acupuncture called Master Tung's Acupuncture. Although he died in 1975, his system lives on through disciples around the world who continue to practice and teach his techniques. (One such disciple was the remarkable Dr. Miriam Lee, whom you can read about in the section "Still illegal but highly effective," earlier in this chapter.)

Although I'm not certified in Master Tung's Acupuncture, here are some of what I know through reading and continuing education about it. This system:

>> Has its own channels, diagnostic methods, and needling techniques separate from the standard acupuncture system.

>> Utilizes the Five Elements theory, but not the 14 channels associated with the organ pairs (see Chapter 2 for discussion of these elements of TCM).

>> Incorporates standard acupuncture points but defines *points* as areas or regions, rather than specific locations.

>> Is highly regarded by TCM practitioners for its simplicity, efficiency, ease of use, and clinical efficacy.

AUTHOR SAYS

When I managed the Doctoral program at my TCM college, Master Tung's Acupuncture was part of the curriculum because it was for advanced practitioners. Studying Master Tung's Acupuncture is one of my professional aspirations.

Making the old new again: Tan Balance Method

The *Tan Balance Method* is a modernized version of acupuncture principles rooted in the *I Ching* (translated as *Book of Changes*), a fundamental text in two ancient Chinese belief systems:

» **Confucianism:** Focuses on personal ethics and morality

» **Taoism:** Focuses on living simply and honestly, in harmony with nature

A central tenet in the *I Ching* (and Chinese philosophy, overall) is balance.

Like many Chinese arts (cultural, martial, and healing), generations of masters passed down the Balance Method over thousands of years. One modern master was Dr. Chao Chen, who attended acupuncture classes at night and worked as a mechanical engineer during the day. Through his studies of the classics, Chen realized the *Nei Jing* was based on the principles of the *I Ching*, and thus, his I Ching Acupuncture was born, integrating all aspects of acupuncture with *I Ching* theory, as well as incorporating concepts from his engineering background. Chen's system was highly influential in the development of balance method styles in Taiwan, Korea, and Japan, and eventually, the West.

The Tan Balance Method, which the late Grandmaster Dr. Richard Teh-Fu Tan developed, was likely influenced by I Ching Acupuncture. Tan studied and apprenticed with several Chinese Medicine masters while growing up in Taiwan. Like Chen, Tan was an engineer, receiving his bachelor's degree in Taiwan and his master's degree in Texas.

In the U.S., Tan noted the frustration of acupuncture practitioners with the lack of immediate and effective clinical results. Based on his understanding of the classical texts, such as the *Huang Di Nei Jing*, Master Tung's Acupuncture, and I Ching Acupuncture, Tan devised his Tan Balance Method to share and teach methods that could yield instant and lasting improvement in patient conditions.

Examining Western Adaptations of TCM Techniques

There are two basic techniques for inserting needles: freehand and guide tube. Freehand is exactly what it sounds like, where the practitioner inserts the needle without a guide tube.

A guide tube is like a sheath for a sword. It's a clear, plastic, open-ended tube that the needle sits inside, with the handle sticking out. The practitioner will place the guide tube with the needle on the point and tap the handle to insert the needle.

Some practitioners prefer freehand for better accuracy and freedom of movement, while others prefer the guide tube for more safety and stability.

I'd have to go very far back in time to find out who first thought sticking needles in the body was a good idea (although historians agree that person was definitely from ancient China). Although acupuncture certainly was the precursor for Western medical acupuncture, dry needling evolved from *injection therapy* (using an injection to treat musculoskeletal pain) on a somewhat parallel track to Western medical acupuncture.

Dry needling

Dry needling gets its name because the practitioner doesn't use the needles to inject a substance into the body. The needles aren't hollow in the way a hypodermic needle is; they're solid and thin, similar to acupuncture needles. Dry needling's history is shorter than acupuncture's by about 2,900 years.

TECHNICAL STUFF

In an article tracing the history of dry needling, published in the *Journal of Musculoskeletal Pain (JMP)* in 2014, the practice of needling without the injection of a substance for pain management was first mentioned in 1941. Later, the term "dry needling" appeared in a 1947 *Lancet* paper in which the injection of pain medication was compared to a saline injection and dry needling. According to the JMP article, interest in the use of dry needling waxed and waned until the early 2000s as research in myofascial trigger points (tender spots in muscles and surrounding connective tissue (fascia)) broadened, and the practice moved toward using acupuncture needles instead of hypodermic ones.

Table 4-1 answers questions that you may have about the similarities and differences between dry needling and acupuncture.

TABLE 4-1   **Distinguishing Acupuncture from Dry Needling**

Elements of Treatment	TCM Acupuncture	Dry Needling
Kind of needles used	Thin, single-use, sterilized, disposable	Thin, single-use, sterilized, disposable
Other equipment	A device that delivers low-level electric current to needles *Moxa* (an herb in stick or loose form) to heat needles	A device that delivers low-level electric current to needles
Insertion points	In specific locations on the body, determined by a practitioner's diagnosis of a patient's condition	In myofascial trigger points, based on where a patient's pain is felt and where it originates
Depth of insertion	Various depths, depending on the condition and the point locations determined by diagnosis	Superficial: 0.2–0.4 in. (5–10 mm) Deep: Under the fat layer to the muscle, which depends on the person. The average range is 0.4–1.2 in. (1–3 mm)
Provider (assuming the practitioner has met the educational and licensing/certification requirements in their state)	Only licensed acupuncturists	Licensed acupuncturists and certified medical doctors, osteopaths (medical doctors who also use hands-on, manual therapy), nurse practitioners, physical therapists, and athletic trainers
Basis of approach	TCM theory and diagnostics (see Chapter 2)	Western medicine theory Evaluation of pain and posture patterns, as well as faulty movements Orthopedic (medical specialty dealing with the musculoskeletal system) testing
What it treats	A full range of chemical, hormonal, mental, reproductive, and musculoskeletal systems in the body	Muscle tissue to reduce pain, inactivate trigger points, and improve movement
Availability	All 50 states and the District of Columbia (but 3 states don't regulate it)	37 states and the District of Columbia

Western medical acupuncture

Western medical acupuncture is an adaptation of acupuncture that medical doctors and doctors of osteopathy practice by using the same type of sterile, single-use, disposable needles that licensed acupuncturists use. They apply their Western medical knowledge of anatomy, physiology, and pathology, and follow the principles of evidence-based medicine. Depending on the level of training that they pursue in other aspects of TCM, Western medical acupuncturists may use TCM techniques other than acupuncture and treat a wider range of conditions, not just musculoskeletal pain. However, they may focus on conditions for which the most supportive research has been done in relation to acupuncture, such as cancer, diabetes, depression, migraines/headaches, and smoking cessation.

Most physicians can practice acupuncture within the scope of their medical licenses. Ten states require physicians to complete a specified number of hours in acupuncture instruction in addition to maintaining a current medical license if they want to practice Western medical acupuncture.

For more about Western medical acupuncture, you can visit the website of The American Academy of Medical Acupuncture, the professional organization of MDs and osteopaths that promotes the evidence-based integration of medicine and acupuncture: https://medicalacupuncture.org.

IN THIS CHAPTER

» **Releasing symptoms with moxibustion**

» **Discovering herbal formulas**

» **Eating to improve your well-being**

» **Using TCM tools in therapy**

» **Moving with tui na, Qigong, and tai chi**

Chapter **5**

Examining Other TCM Therapies

Traditional Chinese Medicine (TCM) encompasses various therapies that can do a reasonable job on their own but produce optimum results together. The most well-known TCM therapy is acupuncture (which you can read about in Chapter 4) — the insertion of fine, sterilized needles in specific locations on the body to stimulate healing. In this chapter, I introduce you to the other TCM therapies that are often used with acupuncture to support recovery and wellness.

Like acupuncture, all but one of the therapies discussed in this chapter are manual therapies, meaning they require hands-on delivery of the therapy by a practitioner or by you, yourself. These are moxibustion, cupping, gua sha, tui na, and the two movement therapies of Qigong and tai chi. The non-manual therapy is Traditional Chinese Herbs (TCH), which requires the acumen of a practitioner to prepare and the cooperation of a patient to consume.

As with acupuncture, TCM principles and theory (see Chapter 2) guide how, where, and when these therapies should be used. Other similarities to acupuncture include their safety (low to no risk of serious side effects) and efficacy (positive outcomes are more likely than not, especially after several treatments). If needles aren't your cup of tea, you may be happy to know that some of these other therapies can be used instead.

All TCM practitioners in the U.S. perform acupuncture, but some may specialize in a specific therapy, such as Traditional Chinese Herbs (TCH), tui na, or gua sha. Depending on how a patient's symptoms present at that moment, a practitioner may apply one or more of these therapies as treatment.

AUTHOR SAYS

I based the information in this chapter on my personal experience in clinical practice, my continuing education courses, and research conducted for this book. Because I often see people new to acupuncture and TCM, I stick to the basics (acupuncture) first, and then I add appropriate therapies in future sessions. If you're curious about a specific therapy, ask your practitioner whether they use that one. However, the practitioner recommends which therapy, or combination of therapies, best addresses your chief concern, and you decide together how best to proceed.

TIP

If you want to know more about herbal treatments specifically, look for TCM practitioners who have a Chinese Herbology certification from the National Certification Commission for Acupuncture and Oriental Medicine (NCCAOM). Some practitioners maintain both a state and national license. Check your state board database to confirm a practitioner's license is in good standing, and ask them about their herbal experience when you call to inquire about their services. Check out Chapter 3 for more licensing information.

Warming with Moxibustion

Moxibustion involves supplying heat, either directly or indirectly, by burning the herb *Artemisia argyi* — that's Chinese mugwort to me and you — over a single acupuncture point, group of points, or area. A practitioner can use moxibustion as a single therapy, but they nearly always use it in tandem with acupuncture. (Flip to Chapter 4 for information on acupuncture.)

REMEMBER

Moxibustion and acupuncture are like peanut butter and jelly — one is rarely mentioned without the other. For example, the textbook that is the basis of licensing examinations at the state and national level is titled *Chinese Acupuncture and Moxibustion* (see Chapter 3 for more about licensing), and my theory course textbook was titled *Fundamentals of Acupuncture and Moxibustion*. The *Huang Di Nei*

Jing (the classic Chinese medical text that is the foundation of TCM, which you can read about in Chapter 4) states, "The present generation should hold in awe acupuncture and treatment with moxa, which cure the diseases of the body."

In the following sections, I discuss the healing properties of moxibustion on the body.

Defining a mothering herb: Mugwort

Cultures around the world use over 500 species and subspecies of *Artemisia* medicinally. Romans in the Middle Ages believed mugwort (which they called "the mother of all herbs") protected people from fatigue and sunstroke. In Europe, people use mugwort tea as a tonic and a digestive aid. In India, people use it to ease cough, anxiety, spasms, and constipation; and to prevent abortion and menstrual problems. The Chumash people, an Indigenous tribe in Southern California, use mugwort for women's health issues such as menopause, premenstrual syndrome, and painful menstruation, not to mention as a calming and dream-inducing agent.

Chinese mugwort is a specific species unique in its use for moxibustion in TCM. Ancient texts and present-day textbooks describe Chinese mugwort as having the following medicinal properties:

>> **Warms the womb and stops bleeding:** Making it particularly suited for prolonged menstrual bleeding or calming a restless fetus to prevent miscarriage. Its warming property also helps treat infertility.

>> **Disperses cold and alleviates pain:** If you have ever had frostbite or felt brain freeze eating ice cream too fast, you know cold pain. This herb effectively counteracts cold-related pain.

>> **Eliminates dampness (*refers to moist conditions that are conducive to rashes and other skin irritations*) and stops itching:** You can use it to treat various skin issues when you apply it as an external wash.

When you dry and burn its leaves, Chinese mugwort becomes *moxa* (the form of the herb used for moxibustion), and its warming action intensifies and creates a deeply penetrating warmth. Practitioners can use moxa in loose-leaf form. When shredded into wool, it can be shaped into cones or rolled into an elongated cigar or stick shape. Modern forms include chalk-like smokeless moxa and premade cones of different sizes.

Burning moxa

In my experience, moxibustion strengthens or boosts the therapeutic action or effect of acupuncture points and helps with chronic conditions such as arthritis, diarrhea, water retention, impotence, back and stomach pain, and stroke. The limited research available shows the radiating nature of its heat affects both shallow and deep skin tissue and activates *thermoreceptors* (nerves that detect and respond to changes in temperature) and *polymodal receptors* (nerves that respond to multiple stimuli, such as heat, pressure, or chemicals).

Although practitioners may burn moxa directly on the skin as the delivery method, there is the risk of burning a patient or blistering their skin. I prefer to use safer methods of providing moxibustion treatments, such as:

TECHNICAL
STUFF

>> **Passing the lighted moxa stick over the target acupuncture needle or area (see Figure 5-1).**

Practitioners can use various stick movements — such as stroking, pecking, circling, and so on — to deliver the heat, resulting in varying levels of temperature and intensity felt by the patient. Because each patient's sensitivity to heat is different, the practitioner asks the patient to let them know if it becomes too hot.

>> **Attaching moxa wool to the acupuncture needle shaft and lighting that wool (see Figure 5-2).**

In this method and the preceding method, the metal of the needle acts as a conduit, so the heat penetrates deeper than a heating pad in areas where you can't fit a heating pad or a heating pad can't effectively treat the problem.

>> **Placing loose leaf or moxa wool inside a moxa box.**

These boxes come in various sizes and shapes (see Figure 5-3). The moxa-in-a-box covers a larger area than heating needles individually. This technique also allows the practitioner to administer other therapies or briefly leave the patient to relax and rest.

>> **Placing a moxa cone (see Figure 5-4) on top of a slice of ginger or garlic resting on the skin.**

The slice acts as both a barrier to protect the skin and as a therapeutic aid: Ginger increases the warming effect of the moxa and improves circulation, while garlic helps relieve swelling and pain.

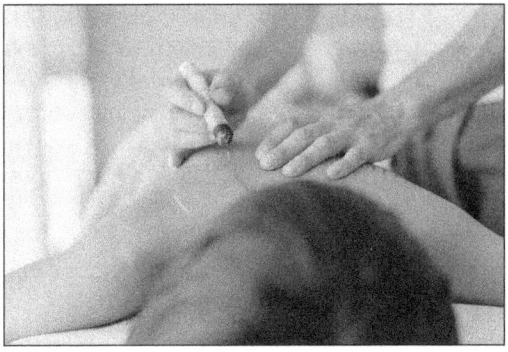

Samuel Perales/Adobe Stock Photos

FIGURE 5-1:
The practitioner heats needles with a moxa stick.

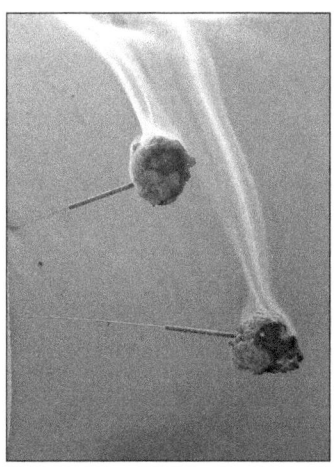

Eugenio/Adobe Stock Photos

FIGURE 5-2:
Moxa wool is shaped into cones on the needle handle and then lit to deliver heat.

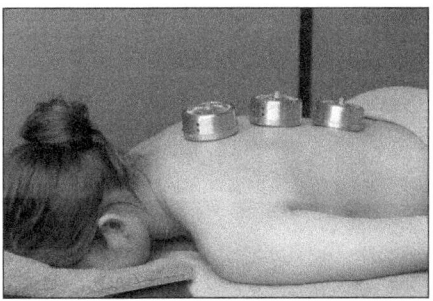

triocean/Adobe Stock Photos

FIGURE 5-3:
Moxa wool or short moxa sticks are put into boxes or containers that are placed on the body.

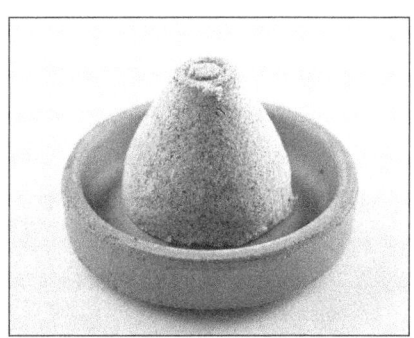

mnimage/Adobe Stock Photos

FIGURE 5-4:
Pre-shaped moxa cones come in different sizes and can be used in a variety of ways.

Using Medicinal Herbs

Around the same time that ancient TCM physicians and scholars organized acupuncture and moxibustion into a healing system, herbs and other *materia medica* (books written about pharmacology) underwent a similar assessment and analysis by other TCM physicians and scholars. The seminal work in this branch of TCM is *Discussion of Cold Damage (Shang Han Lun)*, written by Zhang Zhong-Jing sometime at the end of the Han dynasty (around 220 BCE). Before this text, the mythical Shen Nong wrote the *Divine Husbandman's Classic of the Materia Medica (Shen Nong Ben Cao Jing)*, which was the first book to describe individual herbs. However, *Discussion of Cold Damage* is the source of all TCM prescription manuals that followed it.

Over the centuries, knowledge and literature about medicinal herbs and other natural substances grew while TCM physicians and scholars added new herbs and substances to the *materia medica,* including those originating in other parts of the world, such as Southeast Asia, India, the Middle East, and the Americas. TCM physicians and scholars also reevaluated existing herbs for new applications (similar to doctors using antihistamines, generally used to treat allergies, to also treat insomnia in Western medicine). All the while, TCM physicians and scholars carefully observed and recorded the effects of the herbs individually and in combination. It was just a matter of time before the two branches of treatment (acupuncture and herbs) came together in their theories and concepts to become a system of medicine that has survived for thousands of years and that the scientific community — both East and West — continues to study, adapt, and advance.

PRACTITIONER REFERENCES FOR TRADITIONAL CHINESE HERBS (TCH)

Western TCM practitioners use the book *Chinese Herbal Medicine: Materia Medica, 3rd Edition* (Eastland Press) — compiled and translated by Dan Bensky, Steven Clavey, Erich Stöger, and Andrew Gamble — as their go-to reference text. At just over 1,300 pages, the book examines 480 common herbs and natural substances used to treat numerous conditions and ailments. (It weighs enough to use for bicep curls, if you can fit it in your palm.)

Modern references used in China are more comprehensive. The *Encyclopedia of Traditional Chinese Medicinal Substances (Zhong Yao Da Ci Dian)*, published in 1977 by the Jiangsu College of New Medicine, contains 5,767 entries. It represented China's *materia medica* until the College published its successor, containing almost 9,000 entries — the 10-volume *Chinese Materia Medica (Zhong Hua Ben Cao)* — in 2002.

Looking at food as medicine

The quote "let food be thy medicine and medicine be thy food" is often attributed to the Greek philosopher and designated "Father of Medicine" Hippocrates (460–375 BCE), but scholars have found no evidence that he ever wrote or uttered the phrase. He did, however, write in *The Art,*

> The most famous doctors cure by changing the diet and lifestyle of their patients, and by using other substances. Such capable doctors have the knowledge and ability to use the therapeutic properties of most natural or artificial products.

In accordance with the principles discussed in Chapter 2, TCM practitioners combine the therapeutic properties of individual TCH to create formula prescriptions (or recipes) that address not only a patient's symptoms, but also the underlying cause of their ailments. Just like you can find a basic recipe for chicken noodle soup, TCM practitioners have a basic TCH formula for a cold. However, every cook can put their own spin on chicken noodle soup by changing ingredients or adjusting the ratio of one ingredient to another.

Similarly, a TCM practitioner can start with a basic formula to treat a cold and adjust it, for example, for a patient who has a runny nose and congestion but no fever. The practitioner can adjust it again for a patient who has a high fever and sore throat but isn't constantly clutching a tissue.

Examining the therapeutic properties of TCH

Over the centuries, physicians and scholars documented the therapeutic properties of TCH and came up with formulas, like cookbook authors who develop new recipes. These TCM practitioners noted patients' responses to the treatments and overall results when tweaking their recipes.

While *Discussion of Cold Damage* (see the previous section, "Using Medicinal Herbs") is the foundation of TCH prescriptions, the first comprehensive compilation of herbal properties was the *Materia Medica of Medicinal Properties* (*Yao xing ben cao,* circa 600). This compilation discusses herb combinations, reactions, tastes, temperature, toxicity, function, primary clinical use, processing, and preparation.

The marriage of TCM theory (see Chapter 2) to TCH *empirical* (originating in or based on observation or experience) knowledge wasn't fully realized until medical scholars in the 11th and 12th centuries linked them. In the following list, I describe the five main categories of therapeutic properties to help you get a sense of the intricacy of this aspect of TCM.

>> **Temperature:** As noted in Chapter 2, temperature is one of the fundamental balances that a practitioner needs to achieve through any treatment. The *Nei Jing* (the classic Chinese medical text that is the foundation of TCM) notes, "Hot diseases must be cooled, cold diseases must be warmed."

The temperature properties of TCH include hot, cold, warm, cool, and neutral. One simple example is to use a cold herb to treat a fever. For a mild fever, a warm herb may be the better option. For someone with frostbite, a very hot herb may be selected.

>> **Taste:** In *Chinese Herbal Medicine: Materia Medica, 3rd Edition* (Eastland Press), the authors describe the significance of taste as two-fold — the herb's effects and its therapeutic functions, based on the classic texts.

For example, the *Nei Jing* (see Chapter 2) states, "Acrid and sweet tastes scatter and are yang; sour and bitter substances drain and are yin; the salty taste drains and is yin; the bland taste seeps and drains and is yang."

The yin and yang character of each taste is important with regard to treatment principles (see Chapter 2) and influences herb combinations (see the next section, "Creating formulas").

The therapeutic functions expand on the effects and are used to distinguish their clinical application:

- *Acrid* (sharp, extremely bitter): Scatter and move

- *Sweet:* Strengthen or augment, harmonize, and moisten

- *Bitter:* Drain and dry

- *Salty:* Purge and soften

- *Sour:* Bind (*hold in* or *hold together*) and prevent, or reverse the abnormal loss of fluids and energy

- *Bland:* Suck out dampness and promote urination

- *Aromatic* (spicy): Penetrate and revive

REMEMBER

Temperature and taste are two highly subjective properties. What feels hot to one person may feel cold to another. What tastes sweet to someone may be bland to someone else. So, the selection of TCH according to temperature and taste can vary widely and requires a full understanding of the patient's condition.

>> **Action:** This category is a broader grouping of therapeutic actions based on theories expressed in *Discussion of Cold Damage* (see "Using Medicinal Herbs") and later formulated by TCM physicians into an organizing structure for TCH during the Qing dynasty (1644–1911). Known as the eight therapeutic

methods (*ba fa*), this structure was first documented in *Medical Revelations* (*Yi Xue Xin Wu*) by the physician Cheng Zhong-Ling in 1732. Over time, the eight methods grew to include more methods to address more conditions.

Chinese Herbal Medicine: Materia Medica, 3rd Edition (Eastland Press), the textbook used to educate Western TCM practitioners, contains chapters using translated traditional terms that reflect the original eight methods:

- Promote sweating
- Trigger vomiting
- Purge (strongly eliminate)
- Harmonize (soothe or facilitate)
- Warm
- Clear (release or resolve)
- Tonify (strengthen or support)
- Reduce

» **Channel(s) entered:** The organ channel (pathway for the flow of Qi related to a specific organ; see Chapter 2 for more about Qi and channels) or section of the body that the herb supports or benefits; also indicates the herb's ability to lead the prescription or formula to the organ channel(s) and focus its effects there.

For example, if a patient has indigestion, an herb that enters the Stomach channel will be included in the herbal prescription.

» **Direction:** How an herb's effects move in the body. TCH that rise and float primarily move upward and outward, while those that fall and sink primarily move downward and inward. As the channels enter, the directional property of an herb can guide a formula to where it can act effectively.

For example, an herb that rises can help move a fever out by releasing heat through the pores, thereby promoting sweating. An herb that falls can assist in reducing wheezing by anchoring the lungs.

» **Principle:** Ties TCH selection back to the fundamental theory of achieving one of the Eight Balances, which you can read about in Chapter 2.

For example, going back to the first category of temperature, heat must be cooled, and cold must be warmed.

Creating formulas

The most skilled TCM practitioners in Traditional Chinese Herbs can prescribe formulas from scratch — selecting herbs from the entire *materia medica* to give their patient a unique formula meant only for them. The patient takes these highly specific formulas until they experience a change in their symptoms and condition, for better or worse. The practitioner then modifies the formula in response to the change, and so on.

People all over the world have used plants as medicine for thousands of years, and many of the drugs used today started as one:

>> **Paclitaxel:** From *Taxus brevifolia;* treats lung, ovarian, and breast cancer

>> **Artemisinin:** From the traditional Chinese plant *Artemisia annua;* combats multidrug-resistant malaria

>> **Silymarin:** Extracted from the seeds of *Silybum marianum;* treats liver diseases

Medical and pharmaceutical scientists have done a lot of research on individual plants or herbs, but few studies have been done on full TCM herbal formulas.

Combination strategies

In addition to considering the properties described in the section "Examining the therapeutic properties of TCH," earlier in this chapter, TCM practitioners must also think about how individual TCHs positively interact when combined. Some of these combination strategies include:

>> **Mutual accentuation:** Two substances whose similar functions/actions *accentuate* (boost) their therapeutic effect.

For example, rhubarb root (*Rhei Radix et Rhizoma; da huang*) and mineral salt (*Natrii Sulfas; mang xiao*) are both purging herbs that can be combined to treat severe constipation.

>> **Mutual enhancement:** Two or more substances whose different functions/ actions *enhance* (improve) their combined effect.

For example, rhubarb root (*Rhei Radix et Rhizoma; da huang*), which is a purging herb, and astragalus root (*Astragali Radix; huang qi*), which is a tonifying herb, can help treat painful, red eyes — rhubarb root eliminates heat while astragalus root strengthens Qi (energy or life force; see Chapter 2).

>> **Mutual counteraction:** Practitioners combine substances so that one substance *counteracts* (reduces or eliminates) the negative effects of another.

For example, the pinellia rhizome (*Pinelliae Rhizoma preparatum; zhi ban xia*) is very good in a formula to help resolve a productive cough, but it is toxic if not processed properly. So, fresh ginger rhizome (*Zingiberis Rhizoma recens; sheng jiang*) is also included in the formula to reduce the toxicity of the pinellia rhizome.

Combinations to avoid involve substances that negate or reduce the positive effects of each other, and substances that increase negative effects when combined but not when used individually.

Ingredients and preparation

As with good food, the quality of the ingredients and the method of their preparation make a huge difference in their effectiveness as TCH. TCM practitioners today know how to access safe TCH; they use herbs safely prepared from properly grown and harvested raw materials and substances.

WARNING

The U.S. Food and Drug Administration doesn't inspect or approve the safety or effectiveness of herbs or supplements before they come to market. So, there's a risk that some herbs may be grown with toxic pesticides; some herbs may be counterfeit; or some substances, such as bear gallbladder, may come from endangered species that are illegal to use. TCM practitioners know the manufacturers and distributors of safe, authentic, and legal TCH, so consulting with a TCM practitioner is the best way to ensure that you're getting the right stuff.

Another aspect of safety that you may not think of is the proper identification of the herb(s) being used. TCM practitioners are taught to recognize and identify TCH, so the correct herbs are included in your formula.

Delivery methods

In Western medicine, people commonly deliver or administer drugs and supplements in various ways, such as in a syringe (like a vaccine), a drinkable liquid (like cough syrup), a topical (like an ointment or cream), a mist (like an inhaler or nose spray), or a pill (like everything from antibiotics to antidepressants). TCM practitioners deliver TCH formulas in slightly different ways that you still may find familiar.

DECOCTIONS

The most common way to take TCM formulas is the *decoction*, a type of concentrated liquid. To create a decoction, you boil and let simmer a prescribed combination of herbs in water, preferably in a nonmetal pot, until you end up with the reduced decoction. TCM practitioners believe this is the best way to deliver the maximum benefits of the formula because they are quickly absorbed and therefore, quickly go to work.

TCM practitioners in the West train to prescribe formulas by using whole dried herbs. Some practitioners have their own TCH pharmacy in their office, so they can collect the herbs in the formula and give them to patients. Others will send a formula prescription to a local or regional pharmacy, where the prescription is filled. The patients can then pay for the prescription online and have it shipped to them.

Directions are provided for preparing the decoction, such as how much water to use for boiling based on the dosage and when to drink the decoction. Herbs can also come in powder and pill form, as discussed in the next section. An example of a decoction formula might look like Figure 5-5.

FIGURE 5-5:
A decoction contains a carefully crafted combination of herbs that includes roots, nuts or seeds, flowers, tree bark, and leaves.

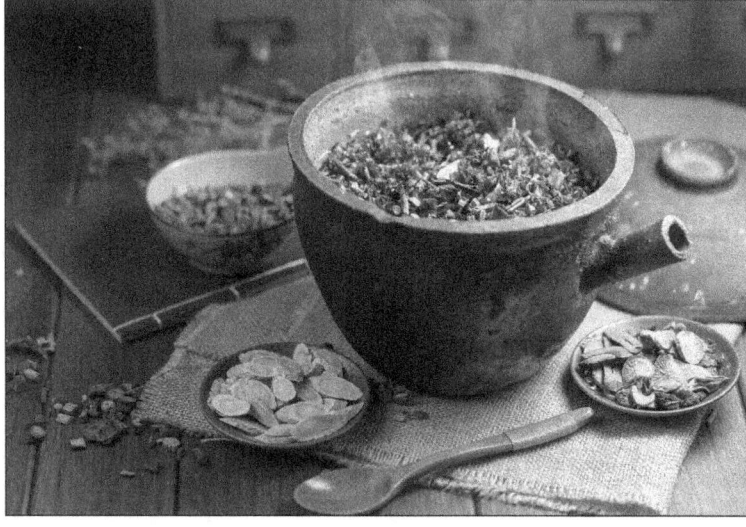

xb100/Adobe Stock Photos

This form of delivery has some downsides:

>> Takes time to prepare

>> Creates a sometimes unpleasant smell

>> More expensive than other methods

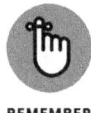

You can also prepare a liquid reduction by using wine or another type of alcohol instead of water, which is referred to as a *tincture* in TCM.

REMEMBER

More recently, TCM practitioners have started offering standard formulas as concentrated liquids in dropper bottles, which can make administration to children or people with difficulty swallowing more convenient. Usually, these are prepared as tinctures (a liquid reduction using alcohol), but can also be prepared as a regular decoction with alcohol added.

AUTHOR SAYS

As much as I want to prescribe decoctions to all my patients, I'm most concerned with them taking the formula. The power of a decoction means nothing if the patient finds the preparation process tedious. (I confess, even I find preparing a decoction tedious.) Some TCH pharmacies receive the prescription, prepare the decoction, and send it to the patient. As with a meal delivery service, this means of obtaining TCH can be very convenient, but also quite expensive. And the decoction can potentially lose potency during transportation.

POWDERS AND PILLS

Two common forms of TCH delivery are powders and pills:

>> **Powders:** Single dried herbs are ground into powder at wholesale manufacturers or pharmacies. Like the dried herbs, TCM practitioners can stock bottles of single herb powders to combine them in the appropriate ratios for formulas, or they can be prescribed and obtained through a local or regional online TCM pharmacy. You can also find standard, already combined formulas (for common or often-encountered ailments) available in powder form. A TCM practitioner can prescribe a *standard formula* (also known as a *patent formula*) or create a tailored version by using individual powdered TCHs. You can stir powdered formulas into warm or hot water, like a tea.

>> **Pills:** Manufacturers place the fine powdered herbs into capsules or mix them with water or honey and a binding agent like rice bran, wheat, or vegetable cellulose to shape a pill. In my experience, TCM practitioners usually administer standard formulas in pill form. I can't think of any time I've seen a pill made with a single herb as the ingredient.

Patients in the West prefer powders and pills over liquid forms of TCH (see the preceding section) because they can take them conveniently and at a relatively low cost. However, as with food, the closer the herbs are to their natural state, the more effective they are. So, decoctions and tinctures are the most potent, followed by powders, and then pills.

AUTHOR SAYS

Alas, I'm not a gifted cook like my late mother or a wiz at whipping up formulas. But I do have a treasure trove of TCH cookbooks that I can reference and master herbalists that I can consult to create and prescribe formulas for my patients with confidence — thanks to the classic masters who laid the foundation and the modern masters who continue to build upon it.

Knowing You Are What You Eat

When it comes to illness, Western and Eastern medicine consider food the source and the solution. You can find some version of the phrase "you are what you eat" in French and German documents from the 1800s that discuss how the food you eat impacts your state of mind and health. But it wasn't until the 1920s that Victor Lindlahr, an American nutritionist, created the phrase we know today for an advertisement: "Ninety percent of the diseases known to man are caused by cheap foodstuffs. *You are what you eat.*"

TCM nutrition theory traces back to the Zhou dynasty (1100–700 BCE), when Chinese high society (rulers, scholars, and the like) considered four groups of healers responsible for medical care:

>> Dieticians for nutrition

>> Internists for internal diseases

>> Surgeons for external illnesses and injuries

>> Veterinarians for sick animals

High society held dieticians, who focused on preventing disease and maintaining health through diet, in high esteem. As one story goes, the pay scale for physicians depended on the continued health of their patients — the lower the number of illnesses, the higher the wages.

As a component of TCM, diet and nutrition play a critical role in preventing and treating disease. The *Nei Jing* (see Chapter 4) states, "When the body is too weak, the therapist should use foods to replenish the deficit." Later, a famous Tang Dynasty physician named Sun Si Miao (618–907) wrote, "Without the knowledge of proper diet, it is hardly possible to enjoy good health."

Modern TCM practitioners combine their understanding of TCM theory with the foods and nutritional knowledge available today. Food and herbs can support or sabotage each other in their effect on the human body. TCM classifies food by the properties of temperature, flavor, organ network, and direction of movement. How food is prepared (boiled, baked, barbecued, and so on) and delivered for consumption (raw or cooked, whole or mashed, for example) also impacts its nutritional benefits. For more on TCM nutrition, see Chapter 11.

Increasing Circulation with Cupping

Cupping involves placing round cups over an area on the body (such as the back, as shown in Figure 5-6) to enhance blood circulation and loosen tight or tense muscles, tendons, and *fascia* (connective tissue). If you watched Michael Phelps swim in the 2016 Summer Olympics in Rio, you may have noticed the rather prominent round bruises on his back, shoulders, and upper arms. Although he (and other celebrities such as Gwyneth Paltrow) may have brought cupping to the attention of the masses, the therapy itself has been used in China (known as *ba guan*), Africa, the Middle East, and Europe for as long as several thousand years.

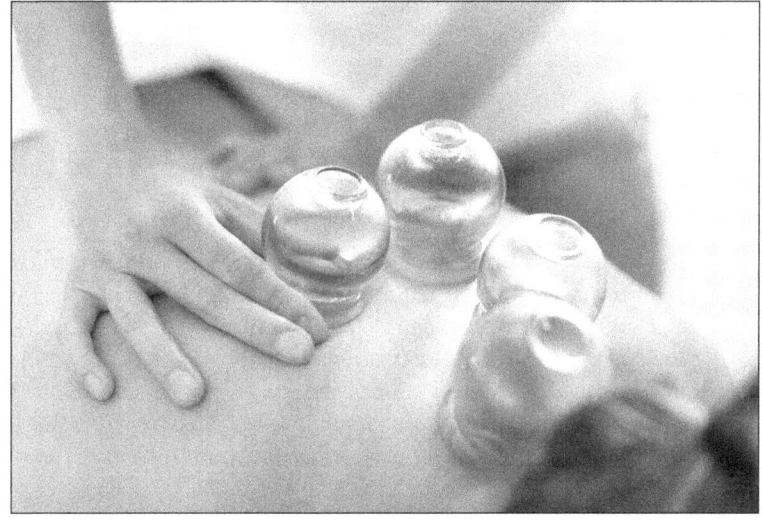

Milan/Adobe Stock Photos

FIGURE 5-6:
The suction from glass cups relieves muscle tension and tightness.

Cupping origins

Early shamans and medicine people used cattle horns as tools to treat boils and abscesses. They placed the base of the horn on the patient (over the area of concern) and sucked the air out through a hole at the point. The idea was to create a negative vacuum and draw the toxins out to the surface layer, where the body would naturally purge them. Historical records indicate cupping was used for everything from tuberculosis and chronic cough to supplementing surgical procedures.

The effects of cupping may correlate to the Western theory of counteraction that dates back to the *Hippocratic Corpus* (a collection of about 60 ancient Greek medical treatises or papers), where "no two diseased actions, affecting the general constitution, can go on at the same time, for any considerable period in the same system." With cupping, the first or initial "disease" of muscle pain is released and resolved to address the second "disease" of the bruising being created by the cup suction.

I interpret the "counteraction" theory as a distraction being created — treating one problem by deliberately introducing a new one so the body shifts its attention away from the original, which will then fade into the background.

Cupping treatments

The materials, shapes, and sizes of cups have evolved, as well as their applications. In Greece, Hippocratic physicians used bronze cups, while the rural population used homegrown gourds. Bamboo, glass, and plastic are the norm now — even a jar or drinking glass can work in a pinch. Instead of the practitioner sucking the air out of the cup, as the early medicine men did, modern cupping practitioners create the vacuum with fire (such as lighting a cotton ball soaked in rubbing alcohol and briefing touching it inside the cup to draw out the air) or connecting the cup to a suction pump.

Properly trained practitioners determine how many cups to use, which size(s), where to place them, whether to move them, how much vacuum to create, and when to remove them. Regardless of material or technique, the same basic concept remains — draw out pathogens or toxins that restrict or impede Qi and Blood movement (according to TCM theory, the smooth movement of Qi and Blood is critical to health; see Chapter 2) to restore free circulation and facilitate healing. In basic Western terms, cupping stimulates both the blood and lymphatic systems to work more efficiently.

Some Japanese practitioners have suggested that cupping, in addition to increasing blood circulation, may increase red and white blood cells and neutralize acidic blood. In a small research study, patient blood tests after cupping therapy revealed increased lymphocyte (white blood cell) counts. And given the tool's direct contact with the skin and fascia, it stands to reason that cupping stimulates the nervous system.

Cupping expert Ilkay Zihni Chirali, who has 40 years of experience as a TCM practitioner in Australia and the U.K., has taught, lectured, and written extensively about cupping and its benefits. According to Chirali, cupping can be used to:

>> Treat pain

>> Improve metabolism

>> Improve blood microcirculation

>> Activate the lymph system's toxin elimination process

>> Tone the skin

>> Address conditions involving heat or cold (such as viruses and inflammation)

Although my experience pales in comparison to Chirali and others, I believe cupping offers multiple applications and uses that give good results. It doesn't cost much, and a trained professional can easily administer it. According to Chirali, in the hands of a properly trained and licensed practitioner, cupping can treat muscle and joint pain, inflammatory conditions, facial paralysis, high blood pressure, cellulite (dimpling of the skin caused by fat deposits) and wrinkles, and anxiety (among other conditions) safely without adverse side effects; that is, unless looking like you got a love hug from an octopus for a few days bothers you.

Counteracting Illness with Gua Sha

Like acupuncture (see Chapter 4) and cupping (flip back to the section "Increasing Circulation with Cupping," earlier in this chapter), *gua sha* is a centuries-old treatment used throughout Asia, in Asian immigrant communities, and by East Asian medicine practitioners worldwide. And like many traditional medical practices, Western medicine often dismissed gua sha as folk medicine that didn't have substantial evidence for its effectiveness.

Until I attended TCM school, I had never heard of gua sha. Now, I'm seeing it everywhere as a DIY (do-it-yourself) beauty treatment to create glowing, wrinkle-free skin. Although I appreciate that this incredible technique is catching on, I'd like to share the real depth and breadth of its application.

Gua sha origins

Gua sha could be the East Asian counterpart to the use of friction as a therapy of counteraction (see the section "Cupping origins," earlier in this chapter). In *On the Surgery* (400 BCE), Hippocrates wrote that soft friction relaxes flesh, moderate friction thickens it, hard friction braces it, and repeated friction reduces or thins it.

Here are the literal translations of the Chinese words *gua* and *sha*:

>> *Gua:* To scrape or to scratch

>> *Sha:* Sand; sharkskin; or red, raised, millet-size rash

Specifically in TCM therapy, *sha* refers to two things:

» Blood stagnation or congestion that accumulates in surface tissue, where a patient feels pain or stiffness

» The *petechiae* (pinpoint-sized red spots under the skin) that result from a gua sha treatment

Gua sha treatments

Despite the treatment's translation of "scraping," Arya Nielsen, PhD, says *gua sha* is more accurately described as press-stroking on lubricated skin by using a smooth-edged tool made of metal, jade, or rose quartz. As the Western authority on gua sha and a dedicated practitioner, professor, and researcher for over 45 years, Dr. Nielsen has brought this traditional technique into modern practice through her work across the country and around the world.

A practitioner applies gua sha in repeated, even press-strokes, moving in one direction only — no back-and-forth stuff — following the contours of the body, as shown in Figure 5-7. Of course, you don't apply gua sha to an injured area or to skin that has a rash, acne, moles, or other signs of irritation or injury.

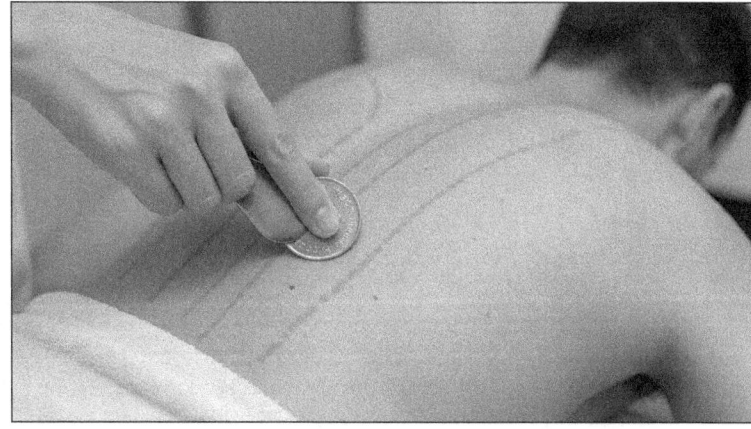

FIGURE 5-7:
Gua sha is administered with a sanitized smooth-edged metal tool (even a coin will do!).

Ispras/Adobe Stock Photos

During treatment, *sha* appear as small red dots that fade in minutes to a blended reddishness. Over a few days, the *sha* disappear completely. Gua sha performs a double duty as a therapy and as a diagnostic tool, similar to cupping (see "Increasing Circulation with Cupping" earlier in this chapter). The color of *sha* and cup marks, and the rate at which they fade, provide important clues to the patient's condition and pace of healing.

Although you may not like the idea of sporting reddish blotches, Dr. Nielsen's vast experience and that of other practitioners and researchers attest to its immense benefits when performed safely and appropriately, which include:

>> Relieving spasms and pain

>> Promoting normal circulation to the muscles, tissues, and organs beneath the area treated

>> Significantly increasing microcirculation in surface tissue

>> Decreasing inflammation

>> Improving mobility

>> Activating the immune system

>> Lowering fever because the raising of sha mimics sweating

A practitioner can use gua sha to treat any illness or condition that causes pain or discomfort, from upper-respiratory issues, such as coughing, to digestive problems, such as indigestion, to pain just about anywhere. Like cupping (see the section "Increasing Circulation with Cupping," earlier in this chapter), gua sha can act as a wonderful add-on or alternative to acupuncture (which I talk about in Chapter 4) or any other TCM treatment.

DIY VERSUS MEDICAL THERAPY

As I mentioned at the opening of this section on gua sha, the technique is being promoted as a DIY (do-it-yourself) treatment, mostly for cosmetic purposes like reducing wrinkles. But tools and techniques that pop up in an online search for gua sha are not TCM medical therapy. Dr. Nielsen refers to those tools and techniques as "gua spa" because they do not elicit sha or follow any TCM diagnostic or treatment principles (see Chapter 2).

As a TCM practitioner, Dr. Nielsen has serious "street cred." Formerly Director of the Acupuncture Fellowship for Inpatient Care at Beth Israel Medical Center in New York City, New York, Dr. Nielsen is currently the Assistant Clinical Professor at the Icahn School of Medicine at Mount Sinai in Madison, Wisconsin. She published the first gua sha textbook and worked with a team in Germany to conduct the first study on the biomechanism of gua sha. As co-chair of the Pain Task Force for the Academic Consortium for Integrative Medicine & Health (see Chapter 7), she contributed to the *white paper* (a document published by authorities on a subject offering

(continued)

(continued)

recommendations) that helped move the needle in changing pain management guidelines in response to the opioid crisis in the U.S.

According to Dr. Nielsen, TCM practitioners also follow safety precautions, which include but aren't limited to:

- Wearing gloves during administration

- Using disposable press-stroking tools, such as a single-use, smooth-edged metal cap (see the accompanying photo) or metal/stainless steel instrument meant to be reused after proper cleaning and sterilization (Jade and rose quartz are used to make tools and rollers for their reputed healing properties, but these tools cannot be used once nor can they be sterilized adequately because they are porous.)

- Using a lubricant such as lotion from a pump dispenser or a balm that they can scoop out of its jar by using a metal spoon for use on a single patient

Metal jar lids or tools, such as those shown in the following figures, can be sanitized. Wood and stone are porous and cannot be sanitized for repeated use.

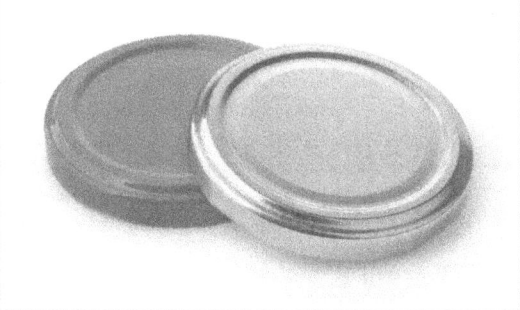

Coprid/Adobe Stock Photos

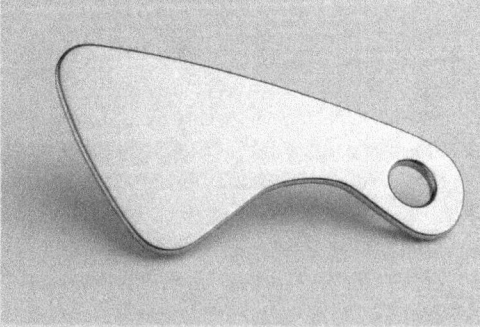

Premium Illustration/Adobe Stock Photos

Incorporating Massage and Movement

Manual manipulation (also known as *massage*) and movement have always been essential elements of well-being, whether they've been acknowledged as such or not. Practitioners of TCM have always considered them essential tools for restoring, encouraging, and maintaining one's health, in the form of tui na (see the following section) for manual manipulation, and Qigong and tai chi (discussed in the section "Moving and breathing for health," later in this chapter) for movement. Each method is an art unto itself that justifies more attention than I can give them in this book, but I definitely want to let you make their acquaintance.

Adjusting with tui na

The key difference between tui na and other manual body therapies is that ancient Chinese practitioners developed it as a medical therapy in keeping with TCM theories and principles. As perhaps the first and oldest documented form of massage in human history (archeological evidence dates back to 2700 BCE), tui na offers time-tested knowledge and techniques for healing hands.

You can translate the phrase *tui na* as "push/pull," "push/grasp," or "hand techniques." As originally intended, practitioners used Royal Style tui na to decrease pain, scar tissue, and *adhesions* (bands of scar-like tissue that form between two surfaces inside the body, causing them to stick together); increase metabolism, range of motion, circulation, and function; and treat soft tissue and joint disorders. Like other tui na styles, it has specific groups of techniques and a treatment sequence.

Tui na, like other manual or massage therapies, can enhance both emotional and physical health. An overview of tui na research discussed in *Braddom's Physical Medicine and Rehabilitation, 6th Edition* (Elsevier), by David X. Cifu, MD, indicates that tui na heals by promoting the metabolism of the manipulated tissue. As a result, the temperature of the tissue increases, which dilates the capillaries and speeds the circulation of blood and *lymph* (a fluid that provides nutrition to cells and tissues and also plays a role in your immunity). This increased blood flow also enhances the supply of nutrients in surrounding muscles and tissue, which promotes growth and development.

The emotional benefits come from an increase in blood circulation, decrease in *cortisol* (a hormone that helps regulate your body's stress response, which can cause a variety of health problems like weight gain and high blood pressure if the body produces too much of it), and increase in levels of *serotonin* (a chemical messenger between your brain and body that plays a major role in mood, sleep, digestion, nausea, wound healing, bone health, blood clotting, and sexual desire, to name a few*)*. Relaxation ensues as muscles and joints loosen, which fosters a feeling of well-being.

TRACING THE LINEAGE OF TUI NA

Like many healing and martial arts, the style of tui na depends on its lineage. I was taught the Royal Style tui na, which has its origins in the Qing Dynasty (1644–1911) and was developed in the Bone-setting Department (*Chuo Ban Chu*) of the Shang Si Yuan Hospital of Orthopedics and Trauma in Manchuria. The Mongolian physicians at this institution provided bone injury diagnosis and treatment for the royal family; hence, it became known as *Royal Style*.

The originator, or 1st-generation practitioner, of Royal Style was Dr. De Shou Tian, who lived sometime in the Qing Dynasty (1644–1911). Royal Style tui na made its way through time and across continents to arrive in the San Francisco Bay Area in the hands of 5th-generation master Xiao (Rocky) Wang, who established a TCM practice in San Rafael, California, and taught at my alma mater, the American College of Traditional Chinese Medicine, from 1995–2003, about seven years before I attended classes there. Before coming to the U.S., he was a medical doctor and surgeon-in-charge at the department of orthopedics and traumatology of Beijing Hu-guo-si TCM Hospital, Beijing, China. As I write this, Wang is still practicing in San Rafael.

One of his students, John Ellis, L.Ac., CMT, PN2, became a 6th-generation Royal Style practitioner and teacher from whom I had the privilege to learn this tui na style. Ellis has a private TCM practice and has taught for over 20 years.

Moving and breathing for health

Ancient and modern medical systems have always associated physical activity with health. The fifth-century Greek philosopher Plato (428–347 BCE) may have said it best: "Lack of activity destroys the good condition of every human being, while movement and methodical physical exercise save it and preserve it."

In the 21st century, researchers have plenty of evidence to prove Plato's statement. A 2020 review of 150 different Cochrane reviews covering 54 health conditions concluded that "exercise reduces mortality rates and improves QOL (quality of life) with minimal or no safety concerns." Another 2023 review published in the *British Journal of Sports Medicine* looked at data from 97 reviews of 1,039 clinical trials involving 128,119 participants. This review found that physical activity "should be a mainstay approach in the management of depression, anxiety, and psychological distress."

In medical research, systematic reviews identify, collect, and analyze research related to health conditions and their associated policies, drugs and drug testing, treatment protocols, surgical procedures and technologies, and lifestyle interventions like diet and exercise. Cochrane reviews are systematic reviews that meet specific criteria to be included in the Cochrane Database of Systematic Reviews, which is maintained by the Cochrane Collaboration (an international, independent, nonprofit network of health researchers, providers, patients, and caregivers). A Cochrane review is considered the highest standard of research in evidence-based health care.

The first unit of the courses I took for the Integrative Health and Lifestyle Program (iHeLp) at the Andrew Weil Center for Integrative Medicine (AWCIM) focused on mind-body medicine (see Chapter 1) and included both physical activity and breathwork. According to Andrew Weil, MD, "Breathing is the bridge between mind and body, the connection between consciousness and unconsciousness, the movement of spirit in matter."

In TCM, movement and breathing come together in the two moving art forms of Qigong and tai chi. Scrolls found in the Mawangdui tombs in China's Hunan province (see Chapter 1) are the oldest documents related to TCM, and they included drawings of exercises for health and pain management (see Figure 5-8). As part of the full complement of tools in a TCM practitioner's toolkit of therapies, I want to discuss them briefly in the following sections.

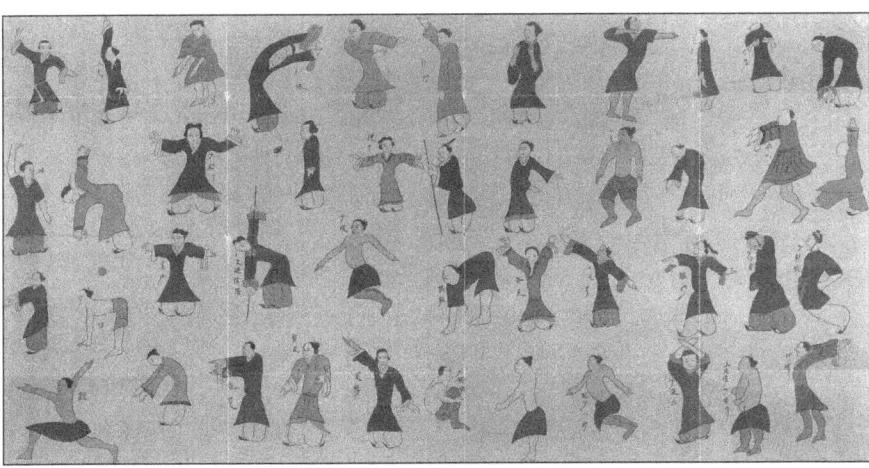

FIGURE 5-8: A reconstruction of an exercise chart for health and pain management, found in Mawangdui Han Tomb No. 3, as displayed in the Hunan Museum.

Qigong

Qigong combines affirmations (positive or motivational sayings or phrases), breath work, meditation, and visualization with movement. In Qigong practice, breath is the vital life force or Qi (see Chapter 2), a belief that seems to relate to the concept of bioelectricity in the body. By practicing Qigong, you can develop the ability to control the life force to prevent disease, promote self-healing, and increase longevity.

Like tui na, long lines of teachers and students passed down Qigong forms and styles. These forms and styles fall into one or more of three main categories:

>> **Medical Qigong:** To heal oneself and others

>> **Martial Qigong:** For physical development and prowess

>> **Spiritual Qigong:** For enlightenment

Most forms and styles emphasize the following:

>> Slow, deep, and long abdominal breathing with breath patterns changing in cadence with movement

>> Fluid and gentle movements performed in a choreographed sequence

>> Focused and disciplined mental awareness and visualization

You stand for active Qigong and move your whole body from head to toe. You can practice passive Qigong like meditation in any position that supports mental focus and breath control. I've even practiced Qigong sitting in the car at rush hour. Some medical qigong practices include self-massage, such as on the abdomen, to promote digestion.

AUTHOR SAYS

I practice two styles, Wild Goose (*Da Yan*), which is more spiritual in nature, and Swimming Dragon (*Taiyi You Long Gong*), which is more martial.

>> **Wild Goose Qigong:** Originated among Taoist monks in the Kunlun Mountains in western China. The form emulates the movements of the wild geese that the monks observed there.

>> **Swimming Dragon Qigong:** Legend has it that a Taoist monk who didn't have much space to exercise in prison developed this style of Qigong. With the water dragon (as seen in the 2021 movie *Shang-Chi and the Legend of the Ten Rings*) as his inspiration, the monk created small, sinuous movements that a person can practice almost anywhere.

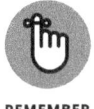

Qigong has been shown to provide the following benefits:

» Increase the exercise capacity of people who are out of shape or are mostly sedentary

» Decrease symptoms of depression; reduce inflammation; stabilize blood sugar

» Reduce musculoskeletal pain

» Improve quality of life and sleep

» Help speed recovery from illness or surgery (when paired with other medical therapies)

Tai chi

Tai chi (or more formally *tai chi chuan,* which translates to "grand ultimate fist")developed as both a martial art and healing art that combines sequences of choreographed movements with deep breathing to foster *Qi* (energy) in the body and promote mind-body harmony. You're probably familiar with the stereotypical image of elderly Asians practicing tai chi in a park. (That stereotype seems like evidence that tai chi practice helps those elderly folks still move so well.)

Research indicates that tai chi has multiple central and peripheral nervous system effects, mainly influencing the immune system and the autonomic nervous system (which regulates breathing, digestion, and heart rate). Other research shows that performing tai chi reduces heart rate, improves *tissue perfusion* (the passage of bodily fluids, such as blood, through the circulatory or lymphatic system to an organ or tissue), and decreases inflammation. Practicing tai chi also enhances neurological function (through the release of adrenaline and endorphins) and strengthens the musculoskeletal system (by encouraging antioxidant activities in the body, which helps to protect cells).

With these effects, the evidence-based health benefits of tai chi include reduced occurrence of and symptoms from falls, osteoarthritis, Parkinson's disease, chronic obstructive pulmonary disease (COPD), cognitive dysfunction, depression, cardiovascular disease, cancer, fibromyalgia, PTSD and other anxieties, hypertension, and osteoporosis. According to *Braddom's Physical Medicine and Rehabilitation, 6th Edition* (Elsevier), by David X. Cifu, M.D., medical programs commonly use tai chi as a standard rehabilitative practice, rather than a complementary or adjunct one.

Both Qigong and tai chi provide a TCM practitioner with routines and practices to improve their own well-being. Most TCM training programs include instruction on these movement styles to set practitioners on the path to not only help others, but also to help themselves.

To find out how you can incorporate tai chi into your health and wellness plan, check out *T'ai Chi For Dummies* by Therese Iknoian (published by Wiley).

Chapter **6**

Knowing What to Expect from TCM Treatment

C onsider your first experience with anything — attending school, starting a new job, having a romantic relationship, welcoming a newborn. During that experience, how did you feel? A little nervous? Kind of excited? Possibly scared? There's not always a first time for *everything*, as the saying goes. But I believe there should be enough first times to keep life interesting, expansive, and fulfilling or rewarding in some way. Perhaps your reasons are similar for considering TCM as a potential approach to self-care — to broaden your health-care horizons, engage with new options, and improve your well-being.

In this chapter, I guide you through a Traditional Chinese Medicine (TCM) treatment. A simple how-to manual can be a helpful resource regardless of whether you're preparing for your first or your tenth experience with TCM because the treatments (and sometimes the experiences) are different for each person each time. In this chapter, I intend to ease your nerves without dulling the sense of discovery and accomplishment that comes with your (maybe first) TCM treatment.

Determining Your Diagnosis

As in any medical setting, the first step of TCM treatment involves trying to figure out what went wrong by getting a diagnosis. Like your doctor, the TCM practitioner will assess your symptoms and identify the disease or condition that caused them. After a diagnosis, you next need to determine how your condition developed by uncovering its *pathogenesis* (the origin and development of a condition).

REMEMBER

Like Western medical professionals, TCM practitioners need to determine what went wrong and how it got that way before they can decide on a course of treatment that can provide the best outcomes. Unlike Western medical professionals, TCM practitioners make this decision by identifying patterns of imbalance that could be the potential cause of your current condition. Please see Chapter 2 for more on TCM theory and concepts.

As discussed in Chapter 2, being healthy essentially means that you're in a state of balance. The eight imbalances that I introduce in Chapter 2 can occur in any combination of vital substances (Qi, Blood, and other vital substances), organs, and channels in your body. TCM looks at these unbalanced combinations as patterns of behavior (or rather, misbehavior), where the normal behavior of your body and its systems has been disrupted or damaged.

TCM practitioners use their ability to distinguish one thing from another — like in *Sesame Street's* "One of These Things" segment — to tell the difference between health and disease, as well as between different diseases. In TCM, the practitioner examines you physically and interviews you about your symptoms to figure out which substances, organs, and channels are involved and how they are out of balance.

I know, it seems complicated. So, to illustrate, consider the common cold, which has the following reported symptoms:

>> Stuffy and/or runny nose

>> Sneezing

>> Sore or scratchy throat

>> Cough

>> Mild/low-grade fever

In Western medicine, the healthcare provider could diagnose the *common cold.* And in very simple terms, a virus transferred by someone coughing in your face could be the pathogenesis of your symptoms. In TCM, the lungs are closely associated with your respiratory system. A TCM practitioner could determine that the Qi (energy and function) of the Lung organ may be Deficient (weak), or Exterior/Cold (cold from outside your body) may be invading or attacking the Lung channel. (See Chapter 2 for details on TCM concepts and theories.) In TCM, these two scenarios of weak Lung Qi or Cold attacking from the outside represent patterns of imbalance, and the TCM practitioner will work to correct the imbalance.

Determining a diagnosis and discovering the pathogenesis involves solving a mystery where you, as the patient, are both the scene of the crime and the eyewitness; your practitioner is the detective. The TCM approach to solving this mystery has an investigation phase that involves four basic steps, which I cover in the following sections; some steps are similar to Western medicine, and others aren't.

Discussing your health history

Sessions with a TCM practitioner begin — like those with any healthcare provider — by talking about what's troubling you. Typical questions you've probably encountered include:

>> What's your chief complaint?

>> What symptoms did you notice, and when did you notice them?

>> What were you doing when the symptoms started?

>> How long have you been experiencing these symptoms?

>> Have you been doing anything to alleviate symptoms? If so, what makes them better, and what makes them worse?

Some practitioners go further into your health history because past health issues can provide important clues to what ails you in the present. Knowing about prior or existing conditions can also help your practitioner choose treatment options for you. These additional questions may include:

>> What have you done differently lately, or what has changed in your life?

These changes can include new food, exercise, travel, cleaning, and personal care products, relationships, residence, or employment.

>> What medications/supplements are you currently taking?

>> What conditions have you been diagnosed with or do you currently have?

>> What medical conditions have occurred in your immediate family members (mother, father, siblings)?

Answering ten questions

In Western medicine, diagnostic methods often include lab testing (a blood test, for example) and imaging (an X-ray of an injury, perhaps) to determine what your condition is and how it developed. Depending on where a TCM practitioner is licensed (see Chapter 3 for more details about licensure and credentials), they may or may not have access to testing and imaging. You can choose to share with your TCM practitioner the testing and imaging results that you get from your primary care doctor, but TCM practitioners generally can't order these tests. However, practitioners are trained to understand what the lab tests and imaging results mean and how those results can contribute to your diagnosis and treatment plan.

Without these modern tools of investigation, TCM practitioners rely on further questioning. After all, when TCM was developed thousands of years ago, none of these tools existed. My TCM master's and doctorate programs introduced me to the ten questions of diagnosis that help me get a better picture of my patient's current state of body and mind. I use them in my practice, especially during the first session with a patient. The questions involve the major systems in the body, which are:

>> **Circulatory:** Heart, arteries, and veins

>> **Digestive (or gastrointestinal):** Stomach and intestines

>> **Endocrine:** Glands and organs that produce hormones, such as the thyroid gland

>> **Immune:** White blood cells that fight infections

>> **Integumentary:** Skin, hair, and nails

>> **Lymphatic:** Nodes and ducts

>> **Musculoskeletal:** Bones, muscles, and tendons

>> **Nervous:** Brain and spinal cord

>> **Reproductive:** Vagina or penis, and other internal and external organs responsible for fertility and sexual development and function

>> **Respiratory:** Lungs, nose, mouth, and throat

>> **Urinary (or excretory):** Kidneys and bladder

The ten questions that follow cover a range of topics that can help your TCM practitioner pinpoint specific issues and determine your TCM diagnosis:

1. **Do you often feel too hot or too cold?**

   Feeling hot or cold is associated with Yang (for hot) and Yin (for cold) as discussed in Chapter 2. If you feel warm a lot and don't like hot weather (or hot yoga), you might have too much Yang (heat). On the flip side, if you avoid air conditioning (even in Arizona), you might have too much Yin (cold). It's also possible that being warm means you don't have enough Yin to even out your Yang, and being cold means your Yang is too low to keep your Yin in check.

2. **Do you sweat when it's not appropriate?**

   Sweating is a way for the body to control body temperature. We sweat to release heat through our pores and cool ourselves down, like the coolant in our cars that keeps the engine from overheating. In TCM, we interpret sweating when a person typically doesn't (sitting still, for example) or not sweating when a person normally does (such as while running a 5-km race) as signs that something is out of whack with one or more of your organ systems. (See Chapter 2 for more about organs in TCM.)

3. **Do you have headaches or dizziness?**

   Where and when headaches and dizziness occur can help narrow options about where the problem originates. As discussed in Chapter 2, TCM theory associates different conditions and their signs and symptoms with specific organ systems. For instance, a headache at the top of the head usually indicates a Liver issue, while a headache on the forehead suggests a Stomach issue. The severity, frequency, and duration of headaches and dizziness can distinguish between Interior or Exterior, and Excess or Deficient imbalances (again, see Chapter 2).

4. **Do you feel pain, and if so, where do you feel it?**

   Pain is one of the most common reasons a patient visits a TCM practitioner. The pain's *location* (in what part of the body you, the patient, feel it), *quality* (the sensation, or how the pain feels), and *duration* (how long you've felt this pain; either *acute,* meaning it started a few days ago, or *chronic,* meaning it has been bothering you for a few weeks or even longer) provide the practitioner with key indicators for diagnosis and treatment. You can find out more about treating pain in Chapter 7.

5. **How many times a day do you go to the bathroom?**

   Like Western medicine, how the body gets rid of waste through urine and stool tells the TCM practitioner whether the digestive and excretory systems are functioning properly. You may find discussing the color, consistency, frequency, and content of your waste products uncomfortable, but these details provide valuable information to your practitioner.

6. **What do you typically eat?**

It's often said that you are what you eat. Eating and drinking (appetite and thirst) are principal habits that impact your overall health. Everything you take in — solid or liquid, animal or vegetable, natural or manufactured — goes through an elaborate sequence of digestion in which your digestive system sorts and distributes nutrients that your body can use to fuel your functioning as a living being.

In TCM, we view what you eat and drink as being transformed by your organ systems into the vital substances of Qi, Blood, and Body Fluid (see Chapter 2). If this system is out of balance, a domino effect impacts every aspect of your well-being. Depending on the TCM practitioner, you may be asked about your appetite, food preferences and cravings, typical diet and mealtimes, and whether you experience any unusual feelings in your abdominal area like bloating or gurgling.

7. **How satisfied are you with your sleep?**

Sleep is as essential to survival as food and water. In TCM, the quantity and quality of your sleep identify a range of patterns involving the organs, the types of imbalance, Qi, and the vital substances (see Chapter 2). And like Goldilocks, you don't want too much or too little; you want the amount of sleep that's just right for you.

8. **When do you think you have the most and least energy during your day?**

Energy is very subjective and difficult to measure. But a patient's perceived level of energy can provide insight into how well their systems are working overall. Early birds have better energy in the morning, which is a Yang characteristic (see Chapter 2), while night owls are more active after the sun goes down, which is a Yin characteristic (see Chapter 2). Energy levels change throughout the day, so highs and lows are additional clues to what may be going on.

9. **How do you feel about dealing with your current condition?**

Emotions can wreak havoc on the body and mind, as anyone who has devoured a pint of ice cream in one sitting or serenaded someone with a boombox can attest. In TCM, each organ is associated with an emotion (see Chapter 2). Discussing how a patient feels about their general health and/or their specific condition allows the TCM practitioner to assess which organ is impacted.

10. **Do you enjoy having sex?**

TCM regards sexual function and development as mostly related to the kidneys, which are responsible for sexual development and growth (see Chapter 2). So, the answers to questions about a patient's desire for and performance during sex can help determine whether you have a Kidney imbalance and how that imbalance may be affecting other organs.

You may find it weird to talk about things that you think are unrelated to your complaint, such as your bowel movements, when you have elbow pain. But to a TCM practitioner, every sign and symptom provides a clue that helps distinguish one condition from another.

Observing your physical appearance

In Western and Eastern medicine, medical doctors and TCM practitioners develop a keen eye for things that look out of place or unusual (just like detectives do in law enforcement). From the moment a patient enters the office, doctors and practitioners observe the person's movement, posture, body shape, voice, complexion, and affect/manner.

For example, if I observe a patient who has a "little pep in their step," "meat on their bones," and rosy cheeks, and who speaks directly and clearly with an ease about them, I'll view that patient as generally healthy. Alternatively, if I observe that a patient is frail, pale, speaking softly, and moving slowly, I may conclude that the patient is unhealthy. Although these examples are obvious and quite generalized, trained doctors and practitioners use this approach to bring the initial picture of a patient's overall health into focus.

Palpating changes

Palpating refers to feeling or touching a patient's body during a medical examination. Using this technique, TCM practitioners can interpret body temperature, any swelling or changes in size or structure of certain body parts, sensitivity to pressure or tenderness, and tension or rigidity. Some TCM practitioners palpate a specific acupuncture point or along a channel. Others just palpate in the area related to your chief complaint.

Many TCM practitioners also use medical devices to get specific measurements for your temperature, oxygen levels, and blood pressure so that they can gather additional objective data.

Understanding the tongue and pulse

The appearance of the tongue and the feeling of the pulse provide the foundation of TCM diagnosis. Without these two pillars of examination, the patient's picture is incomplete, the mystery goes unsolved, and the jury's out on a recommended treatment. In my experience, examining the tongue and taking pulses helps me to confirm or adjust my diagnosis and treatment plan. Others have elevated this skill into an art, diagnosing patients accurately by tongue and pulse alone.

Inspecting the tongue

A TCM practitioner looks at two parts of the tongue: the tongue body itself and the coat that covers it. Sections of the tongue body correspond to organs (see Figure 6-1), and the practitioner notes colors and shapes that appear there:

>> **Colors:** Include red, pink, purplish, grey, or black. The colors can appear uniformly on the tongue surface or in certain spots, such as the back, sides, or tip.

>> **Shapes:** Cracks, bumps, indentations, and swollen or shrunken areas.

Tongue Reflexology Chart

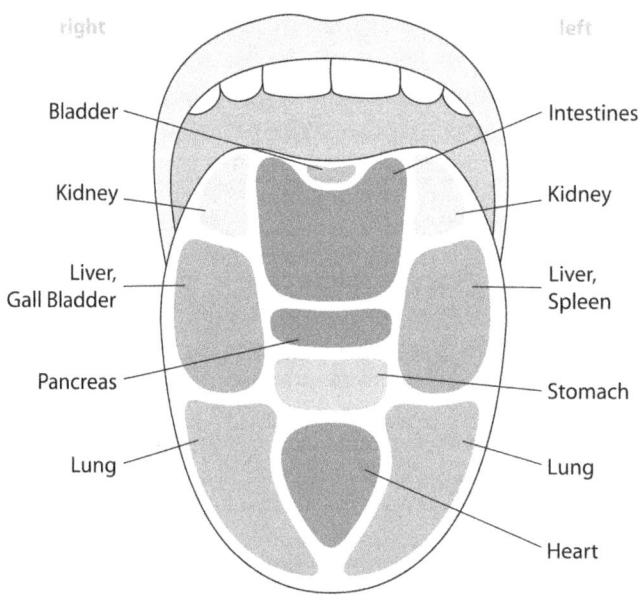

right   left

Bladder — Intestines

Kidney — Kidney

Liver, Gall Bladder — Liver, Spleen

Pancreas — Stomach

FIGURE 6-1: According to TCM, the organs are reflected in different areas of the tongue.

Lung — Lung

— Heart

Peter Hermes Furian/Adobe Stock Photos

Together, tongue colors and shapes help point out imbalances and where they're occurring. For example:

The center of the tongue represents the Spleen and Stomach. It could be pale red, red, or scarlet, which indicates levels of Heat in one or both of those organs, as well as how deeply inside the illness has gone and whether it involves Excess or Deficiency (see Chapter 2).

The *coat* on a tongue is normally a thin, transparent film and is hardly noticeable. The coat reflects how well your digestive system is working and tells a TCM practitioner a lot about what's going right or wrong in your body. The practitioner notices the thickness, color, coverage, and texture of the coat:

>> **Thickness:** A thin coat is usually normal, but can be a sign of Deficiency, while a thick coat is usually an Excess sign.

>> **Color:** White, yellow, gray, black; typically indicates levels of Heat and Cold.

>> **Coverage:** Where on the tongue the coat appears. Even distribution is a healthy sign; a few gaps here and there can indicate Deficiency (see Chapter 2) of some kind.

>> **Texture:** Too moist or puddling can indicate an Excess of Fluids or a Deficiency in Yang (see Chapter 2), while a slick and shiny coat (like oil) can signal Excess Damp, and Cold or Heat, depending on the color. Other textures include a dry, sand-like coat that can signify Deficiency of Yin or loss of Body Fluid due to Excess Heat. A coat that's curdled like cottage cheese may indicate Excess Yang/Heat in the stomach.

Feeling the pulse

Everyone has had their pulse taken at some point by a machine or by touch. In every medical or police drama, someone checks for a pulse to make sure the person is alive. But TCM takes pulses to a different level completely.

A TCM practitioner feels your pulse on both wrists. They place their index, middle, and ring fingers along your radial artery, which runs up the thumb side of your arm, as shown in Figure 6-2.

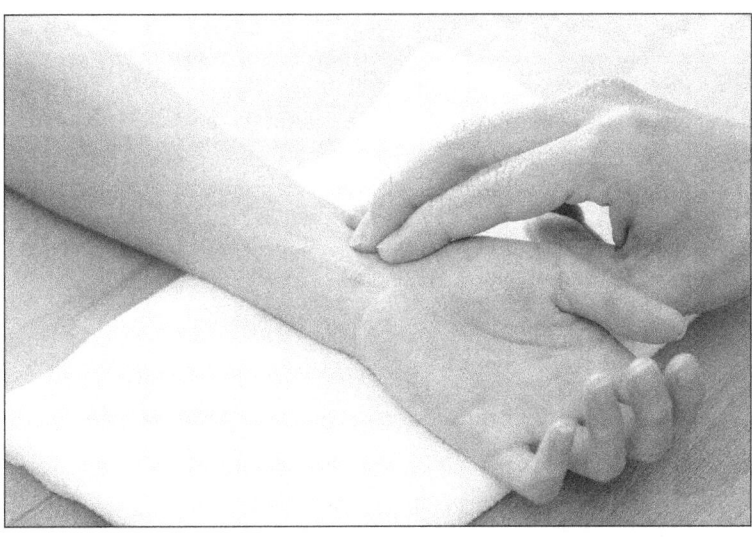

FIGURE 6-2:
Feeling a pulse on the wrist.

leungchopan/Adobe Stock Photos

The position of each of these three fingers on each wrist corresponds to an organ/channel. The practitioner rests their fingers lightly at first, and then gradually applies a little pressure to check your pulse at three depths: surface, middle, and deep. The character of what they feel at each position and each depth amounts to nine pulses that signal the type of imbalance and the organ system(s) involved.

Character refers to what the pulse feels like, meaning the TCM practitioner can determine:

>> Does it feel thin like a thread to indicate a deficiency, thick like a noodle for excess, or tight like a violin string as a sign of stagnation or blockage?

>> Does it bounce up against the fingers for excess or dissolve under their pressure for a deficiency?

>> Does it flow like a wave that surges forward and fades away to indicate excess?

>> Does it feel like a strand of pearls sliding under the fingers as a sign of excess?

Patients can have a variety of character combinations, and it takes a highly accomplished practitioner with seriously sensitive fingers to identify them.

Receiving Treatment(s)

After a TCM practitioner forms a diagnosis, they make a plan for treatment that includes one or more components or techniques (as described in Chapters 4 and 5). You and the TCM practitioner work together to decide how many sessions you need to achieve your goals. The number of sessions you choose often depends on how long you've had your problem. Because a TCM practitioner gears treatment toward restoring balance, how long you've been out of balance determines how long it takes to recover healthy function.

I've seen the benefits of TCM treatment accrue over time, very much like interest on an investment. TCM encourages, coaxes, and reminds the body's ecosystem to heal itself — which the body does by transmitting signals, flipping switches, converting proteins, and performing countless other actions — to return its balance.

Wondering whether it hurts

Before I received acupuncture for the first time, I was nervous. I imagined myself as a pin cushion — or even worse, Pinhead from the *Hellraiser* movies (which I've never seen, but the image is iconic). I was pleased to be so wrong.

Modern acupuncture needles are commonly made from stainless steel, which makes them go in with almost no resistance or pain. They vary in thickness (called their *gauge*) from as thin as a human hair to half the thickness of a sewing needle, as shown in Figure 6-3. For comparison, about 25 acupuncture needles can fit inside a 23–25 gauge (typical sizes for vaccination) hypodermic needle.

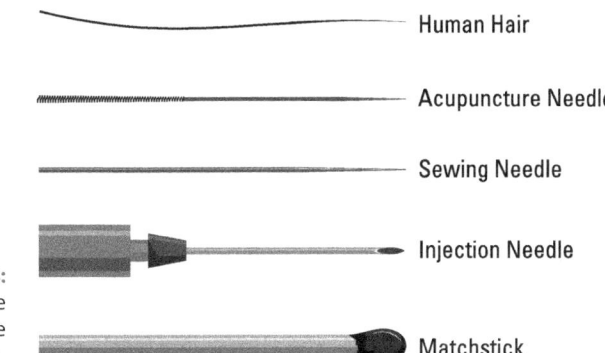

Human Hair

Acupuncture Needle

Sewing Needle

Injection Needle

Matchstick

FIGURE 6-3: Acupuncture needle comparisons.

Needles range in length from ¼ inch up to 6 inches, but the maximum length I've ever seen used is 4 inches. At the top of each needle is either a plastic or steel handle, which the practitioner uses to hold and insert the needle.

The TCM practitioner chooses needle gauge and length based on where they plan to insert the needle (for example, the thigh or the foot) and the size of the patient (such as longer and thicker for larger people and shorter and thinner for smaller people).

Licensed TCM practitioners develop the skill to insert needles with the least amount of discomfort based on thousands of hours of training and practice. Licensure requirements vary from state to state in the United States. But in California, TCM practitioners need to complete no less than 3,000 hours of theoretical and clinical training before they can even take the license exam.

Practitioners' training also identifies how deep you can insert a needle at each of the 300-plus acupuncture points on the body that are part of the TCM curriculum. Rest assured that none of these depths goes more than an inch or two, at most. To read more about acupuncture, see Chapter 4.

Other TCM techniques, such as cupping and gua sha (discussed in Chapter 5), have the potential to cause discomfort or pain. However, this all depends on your chief complaint and TCM diagnosis, as well as the experience and skills of your TCM practitioner.

ACUPUNCTURE SENSATIONS

My first memory of a needle is getting a shot at the doctor's office as a child. Ever after, I dreaded those shots. I can't think of anyone who ever said they liked them. TCM practitioners do everything they can to make your experience nothing like that memory.

As someone who has received and given acupuncture, I can tell you what I've felt and what patients have described to me. At times, I feel nothing except a slight prick from the needle going in. Sometimes, I don't even feel the slight prick, but I sense that something is there. Other times, I feel a zing, like a zipper being opened or closed, starting from the insertion point. On occasion, I feel a whirling twinge at the insertion spot. And sometimes, I feel nothing at all.

Patients have expressed their sensations in the following ways:

- Warmth around the spot
- Heaviness or feeling weighed down
- Tingling
- Lightness
- Electricity

Patients also often describe feeling weirdly calm while on the table or immediately after the treatment. My favorite description from one patient is that she felt "glimmers" of happiness throughout the days following a treatment. This kind of feedback gives me "glimmers."

REMEMBER

Always tell your TCM practitioner when you experience extreme pain or discomfort during your treatments. I tell my patients that whatever they feel is okay, as long as it doesn't hurt, make them uncomfortable, or distract them from the healing purpose of the treatment.

Positioning for treatment

Depending on your chief complaint and subsequent diagnosis, you receive your treatment lying either on your back or on your stomach. In most settings, you lie on a slightly padded table, like the kind used for a massage. The table may be covered with a table-sized heating pad.

If you're on your back, you can rest your head on a pillow (or two) and have a *bolster* (a rounded cushion) under your knees to protect your lower back and keep your legs in a relaxed position. If you're on your stomach, you rest your head in a padded face cradle to support your neck.

After you get settled, the TCM practitioner positions a heat lamp over your feet and legs, or anywhere else you might feel cold. They may also provide sheets and/or blankets if you need an extra layer. I can't speak for all practitioners, but you can ask if these are provided when you call for your first appointment.

If you're in a *community acupuncture clinic* — where multiple patients are treated at the same time, often in a single room, by several practitioners — you likely get seated in a chair or a recliner.

Assuring Your Safety

The primary objective of every healthcare provider is to do no harm and to do whatever is safe and legal within their scope of practice to help a patient. As discussed in Chapter 3, each state in the U.S. has a licensing board that administers testing for licensure and regulates acupuncture practice in that state. Depending on the state, other TCM techniques like cupping (see Chapter 5) are included in the acupuncture scope of practice and, therefore, regulated as such. Also, as discussed in Chapter 3, the National Certification Commission for Acupuncture and Oriental Medicine (NCCAOM) tests for national certification, monitors regulatory developments or changes in individual states, and provides guidance on ethics and patient safety.

At the state and national level, all TCM practitioners must receive training and certification in Clean Needle Technique (CNT) before they can receive a license to practice. The national organization, the Council of Colleges of Acupuncture and Herbal Medicine (CCAHM), manages and administers CNT certification. (See Chapter 3 for more information on CCAHM.)

Using the Clean Needle Technique

Before COVID-19 — specifically, up until March 2020 — the CNT course involved an all-day, in-person session based on CCAHM's *The Clean Needle Technique Manual.* The session ended with a written and practical exam. The practical exam required the potential practitioner to demonstrate CNT procedures for handling, inserting, and throwing away needles.

When CCAHM had to make necessary changes because of COVID-19, the CNT course and certification exam were converted to an online format. At the time

I'm writing this book, the CNT Manual currently in use is the 7th Edition, which was revised in January 2024. (If you're curious, you can download the *Manual* at `www.ccahm.org/ccaom/cnt_manual.asp`.) The post-COVID course includes 16 online sections and an additional 15 hours of recommended reading and studying to prepare for the written and practical exams. The practical exams are conducted via video with an online proctor observing the demonstration.

Following the CNT Manual

The CNT Manual covers all the possible risks associated with acupuncture, moxibustion, cupping, electroacupuncture, gua sha, ear seeds, tui na, and other lesser-known procedures. (I discuss many of these procedures in Chapter 5.) More importantly, the CNT course teaches practitioners how to avoid and/or minimize these risks by providing guidelines for best practices in relation to each technique. One obvious example guideline tells the practitioner to make sure that they remove all the needles from a patient's body before the patient leaves.

The CNT course further emphasizes sanitary processes taught in TCM schools, such as handwashing, maintaining clean surfaces, preparing the patient's skin before insertion, inserting the needle to the proper depth, and removing and safely disposing of needles.

Preventing infections

It's exceedingly rare to get an infection from a TCM treatment. In a systematic research study that reviewed reports from 25 countries over a 12-year period, 239 cases of infection were reported from acupuncture, and 14 adverse events, like burns, were reported from moxibustion and cupping. I'm no statistician, but that seems pretty rare.

By comparison, the Centers for Disease Control and Prevention (CDC) published a survey of 183 U.S. hospitals that reported an estimated 648,000 hospitalized patients who suffered from 721,800 infections.

In any healthcare setting, from hospital bed to dentist chair to a TCM treatment table, it's exceedingly important to minimize the risk of infection. For this reason, CNT certification requires practitioners to know the following:

>> **Infections related to acupuncture and related procedures**

- Hepatitis B and C (blood contact)

- Staphylococcus (skin contact)

- Influenza (airborne)

- COVID-19 (airborne)

>> **Infections in healthcare settings, in general**

- Group A *Streptococcus* (GAS) (mucosal contact)

- Herpes Simplex Virus (HSV) 1 & 2 (skin or mucosal contact)

- Human immunodeficiency virus (HIV) (blood contact)

- Methicillin-resistant *Staphylococcus aureus* (MRSA) (skin contact)

>> **Risks to healthcare workers**

- All of the above

>> **How to prevent infections from being transferred in healthcare settings**

- Handwashing

- Using sterile (where required) or properly cleaned equipment and devices

In a TCM treatment setting, CNT certification makes sure that you and your practitioner are safe and well-informed.

Using needles one time only

TCM practice involves the safety feature of using sterilized, individually packaged needles only once. The practitioner discards the needles in *sharps containers* (red plastic containers specifically used for safe disposal of hazardous objects) that then go to a proper hazardous waste management facility.

Obtaining your consent

Before your first session, your TCM practitioner gives you an informed consent form to read and sign. The informed consent information describes the TCM procedures/techniques that the practitioner may use or offer to you, and the potential risks of those procedures. For the sake of brevity, I've described the risks associated with acupuncture, which include the following:

>> **Minor risks**

- Minor swelling (also applies to cupping and gua sha)

- A little bleeding (also applies to gua sha)

- Discoloration of the skin (also applies to cupping, moxibustion, and gua sha)

- Small bruise (called a *hematoma*) at the site of needling

- Lightheadedness (usually associated with patients who haven't eaten for several hours before treatment)

>> **Major, but uncommon risks**

- Fainting

- Spontaneous abortion

- *Pneumothorax* (a partially or fully collapsed lung caused by air in the chest cavity)

- Infection

Traditional Chinese Herbs (TCH) or nutritional supplements are considered safe in TCM practice. However, like anything you consume, some substances can be toxic in large doses. Some are inappropriate during pregnancy, may interact with medications or other supplements (see Chapter 14), or may have side effects of their own.

Potential risks from TCH include, but are not limited to, allergic reactions, nausea, gas, stomachache, vomiting, headache, diarrhea, rash, hives, and tingling of the tongue. Some possible side effects of applying topical creams, liniments, ointments, and plasters are rashes, hives, and tingling of the skin.

TIP

Carefully read any informed consent forms presented to you, and be sure to ask the practitioner any questions about anything that's not clear.

Knowing when NOT to use TCM treatments

Contraindications (symptoms or conditions that make a particular treatment inadvisable) for acupuncture, other TCM treatments, and certain herbs may include:

>> History of bleeding disorder

>> An implanted pacemaker or prosthetic heart valve

>> Use of certain medications, such as current *anticoagulation therapy* (which prevents the blood from clotting)

>> Pregnancy (depending on the patient's health history, acupuncture is generally safe and supportive of a healthy pregnancy. However, there are specific acupuncture points that should not be used during a pregnancy, and licensed TCM practitioners know what they are. Also, see Chapter 9 on TCM for reproductive health.)

Notify your practitioner if any of these conditions apply to you. And, of course, you can always decline any treatment method that concerns you.

Preparing for Treatment

When I first started my TCM training, the most common place to receive TCM treatment was in a private practice or a community acupuncture clinic. Since then, the accessibility of TCM has expanded and is now offered in public health clinics, hospitals, cruise ships, spas, and integrated medical settings.

In my experience as a patient and a practitioner, you receive several forms before your first appointment. The most typical include:

>> Registration/patient information

>> Informed consent

>> Notice of privacy practices (NPP)

>> Acknowledgment of receipt of NPP

In my practice, I also include:

>> Welcome letter

>> Overview of patient and practitioner partnership

>> Health history questionnaire

>> Patient financial responsibility

>> COVID-19 consent to treat (Accepting and acknowledging the risks of contracting COVID-19 while being treated in a healthcare setting)

TIP

In most TCM treatment settings, you have the option of completing the forms in advance or on-site. I recommend that you complete them in advance because that way, you get more time with the practitioner so that you can discuss your chief complaint and ask them questions about potential treatments.

Knowing what to wear

As I discuss in Chapter 2, you have over 300 points located all over your body that are identified as acupuncture points with therapeutic actions. Because most of my new patients have never had acupuncture or any other TCM treatment before, I prefer to have them lying on their backs for the first session so that they can see me and what I'm doing, and they can ask questions freely.

I recommend wearing loose, comfortable clothing that allows you to roll up your sleeves and pants legs so that the practitioner can access your hands, arms, feet, and legs.

Depending on the weather, you can wear a t-shirt and shorts, or sweatpants and a loose, long-sleeved top. Because you'll be on the table for at least 20 minutes, consider wearing something that you might nap in. Falling asleep happens frequently in my experience, both as a patient and practitioner.

Deciding what to do before and after

I recommend that my patients have a light snack about an hour before their session. TCM treatment activates systems and processes to restore balance in your body, and your body's response is unpredictable. I think of it as fueling up before a workout because your body will be working to respond to what the treatment is asking it to do. (I go into details about how acupuncture works in Chapter 4.)

After your TCM treatment, just like after a workout, drinking plenty of water can refresh and revive you. And if possible, take it easy for 30 to 60 minutes after your treatment to give your body a chance to process and adjust to the treatment.

In the days after treatment, observe how you feel and whether anything has changed so that you can give your practitioner feedback to guide your next treatment.

3

Choosing TCM for the Body and Mind

Understand pain and how TCM can help relieve common pain conditions such as arthritis, low back pain, and headache

Supplement addiction recovery and support mental health with help from TCM

See how TCM improves fertility in men and women and helps maintain a healthy pregnancy and delivery

Make the most of cancer treatment and minimize side effects on the path to survivorship

Chapter **7**

Relieving Pain

P ain is the body's early warning system. It's like the check-engine light on a car's dashboard calling for attention to your body. Ignore it, and you can end up with a hefty repair (um, medical) bill.

Although everyone feels physical pain at one time or another, the experience is entirely subjective and unique to each person. If you're a stranger to chronic pain, hallelujah! You may choose to skip this chapter, though you'll miss some helpful information on pain-management techniques that use Traditional Chinese Medicine (TCM). I provide an overview of pain and how TCM approaches some common conditions.

There are more than 370 International Classification of Diseases (ICD) diagnosis codes associated with pain. In this chapter, I cover a handful of the most common physical pain conditions. I talk about mental and emotional pain in Chapter 8.

TECHNICAL
STUFF

The World Health Organization (WHO) develops and publishes the ICD codes that are used worldwide to code diseases and medical conditions. The U.S. Centers for Disease Control and Prevention's National Center for Health Statistics modifies them for clinical use (ICD-10-CM) in the United States. In addition, the Centers for Medicare and Medicaid Services update and maintain codes for inpatient procedures (ICD-10-PCS).

Please don't use any of the signs or symptoms listed in this chapter to self-diagnose because any number of conditions can cause them. Consult your primary care physician for proper diagnosis and treatment for any symptoms that trouble you.

Defining Pain

Before we move on, I want to offer a primer on pain. The pain I'm referring to in this chapter is physical suffering. As you probably know, you can feel pain for a short time (called *acute*), or it can stay with you for longer (known as *chronic*), for three to six months or more.

Pain gives you a warning that something's wrong. Acute pain has a specific cause, such as getting a splinter in your finger or twisting your ankle. Address the cause — remove the splinter or ice and rest the ankle — and the pain goes away.

Chronic pain usually starts out acute, but even after you eliminate the cause, you still feel pain. Perhaps a small piece of the splinter remains and becomes infected, or you keep playing basketball after the ankle twist. Now, you have a new — potentially more serious — problem that needs attention.

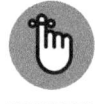

Pain and discomfort are two different things. Don't tolerate *pain*, thinking you can take enough aspirin or you can wait it out. *Pain* is when something hurts so bad that you are unable or unwilling to do regular daily tasks, and you can't focus or concentrate on anything. *Discomfort* comes and goes and doesn't interfere with your life, such as soreness after exercising neglected muscles, carrying groceries up your townhouse stairs, or standing for three hours at a rock concert (all of which have resulted in *discomfort*). Persistent, ongoing (two weeks maximum) *discomfort* can eventually become *pain*, so see your doctor if your *discomfort* goes on too long.

Types of pain

Medical professionals often describe pain as either peripheral or centralized:

>> **Peripheral pain:** An immediate radar ping to the brain; the one that prompts an outburst such as "Ouch!" (or something a little more colorful) and sends you to the medicine cabinet for a pain reliever, or a bandage and antibacterial ointment. See Figure 7-1 for an example.

>> **Centralized pain:** Like a smoke detector that has a low battery — it beeps and then goes quiet, only to beep again some seconds later. You can replace the battery in a beeping smoke detector, but the source of centralized pain in your body may be more difficult to find.

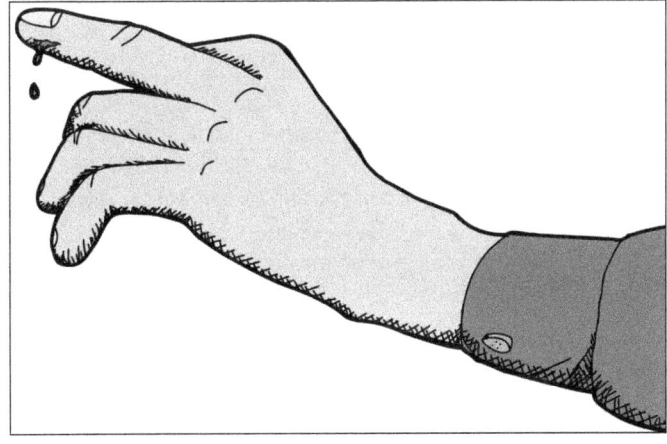

FIGURE 7-1:
Peripheral pain is what you feel instantly when you cut your finger.

Although they don't strictly equate, peripheral pain is typically acute, and centralized pain is typically chronic. You usually experience acute and peripheral pain as temporary annoyances that you can readily resolve. Chronic and centralized pain can leave you with an ongoing source of frustration that sets off a chain of other serious physical and psychological conditions, such as obesity and depression, that significantly reduce your quality of life.

Sensing pain

The intricate workings of the central nervous system go well beyond the subject of this book (and well beyond my area of expertise), but I do want to touch on how the human body is designed for self-preservation. Pain acts as a radar that warns of incoming danger or risk. Many modern cars have sensors that blink and beep if you drive too close to something or if another car occupies the lane beside you. If you ignore those lights and sounds, something bad probably happens.

People have studied how the brain recognizes and communicates pain for ages. The following are classifications for types of physical pain:

>> **Nociceptive:** *Nociceptors* (pain sensors) protect you by registering a *noxious stimulus,* which can cause an alarming level of pain, and trigger an immediate action or reaction to avoid further harm (see Figure 7-2). For example, if you

pull a tray of cookies from the stove, and your well-worn oven mitt brushes against the inside wall of the oven, in a split second, nociceptors detect the heat of the hot metal and transmit a message to your brain that translates to "Danger, Will Robinson!" And you jerk your hand away (hopefully without spilling your cookies on the floor).

» **Inflammatory:** I once severely sprained an ankle playing basketball. It swelled to the size of a softball, turned different hues of black and blue, and had me on crunches for at least a week. It was sensitive to touch and throbbed almost constantly.

The immune system activates this kind of pain (called *inflammatory*) and creates a hostile environment that affects the ankle, foot, and adjacent tissues and bones, encouraging you to avoid movement, physical contact, or further use or stress until your body can safely resolve the injury (or infection). The inflammation and pain served as barriers between my ankle and my desire to get a move on to promote healing and prevent greater injury. See Figure 7-3.

» **Pathological:** This kind of pain isn't protective. It's a short circuit in the nervous system that continues to signal pain after your body heals an injury or infection, or even when your body has no damage at all. For example, a person can become highly sensitive and feel pain from things not usually considered painful, such as the texture of a wool sweater.

REFLEX ACTION OF HAND

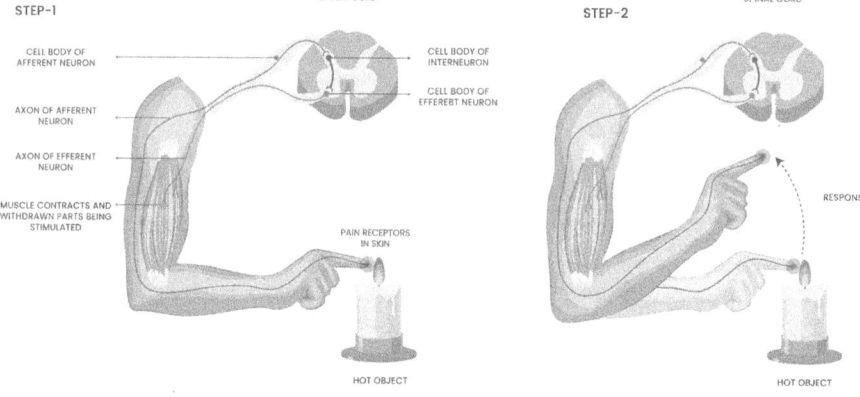

FIGURE 7-2:
Nociceptive pain is an immediate response to a threat, such as heat.

Nandalal/Adobe Stock Photos

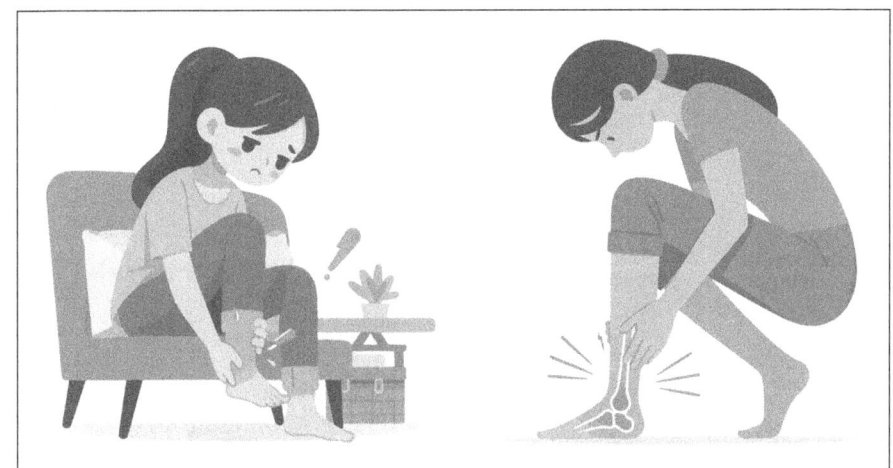

TEGUH/Adobe Stock Photos

FIGURE 7-3: An ankle sprain is a classic example of inflammatory pain.

Considering the mental side of pain

Although pain is a physical sensation, it elicits any number of emotions and thought patterns, such as worry, frustration, depression, a sense of defeat, or even fear. The mental aspects of pain can affect how patients experience, describe, and respond to it. Mental pain can even distort how patients interpret or perceive the sensations that they're experiencing. Emotions can turn up the volume on pain, so practitioners need to consider and treat psychological factors in tandem with the physical ones. Although not specifically tied to pain, Chapter 8 discusses a few mental health conditions that can be treated with TCM.

Knowing the high cost of pain

In addition to the impact pain has on individuals and their families, pain takes its toll on society and the healthcare system. Based on data from the 2016 National Health Interview Survey (NHIS), about 50 million adults in the U.S. suffered from chronic pain. Studies have linked chronic pain to numerous physical and mental conditions, and it contributes to high healthcare costs and lost productivity, estimated at $560–635 billion annually. Sadly, pain — and the overuse of opioids to treat it — has millions struggling with addiction, which has caused an alarming number of overdose deaths from prescription opioids since 2005.

In response to this crisis, resources, research, and collaborative thinking focused on how to best treat acute and chronic pain. Formed in 2016, the Pain Management Best Practices Inter-Agency Task Force within the U.S. Department of Health and Human Services published its Final Report on May 9, 2019. The Task Force report emphasizes "an individualized, patient-centered approach for diagnosis and treatment of pain" and recommends "complementary and integrative health, including treatment modalities such as acupuncture, massage, movement therapies (such as yoga and tai chi), and spirituality, should be considered when clinically indicated."

Reducing Arthritis and Joint Pain

Arthritis and joint pain seem inevitable while you age. In the following sections, I talk about the kind of arthritis and joint pain that comes from repetitive stress, overuse, gradual loss of cartilage, or all of the above. This type of arthritis, called *osteoarthritis,* affects over 32.5 million people in the U.S., according to the Centers for Disease Control and Prevention (CDC). Figure 7-4 illustrates how osteoarthritis can affect a knee joint.

OSTEOARTHRITIS

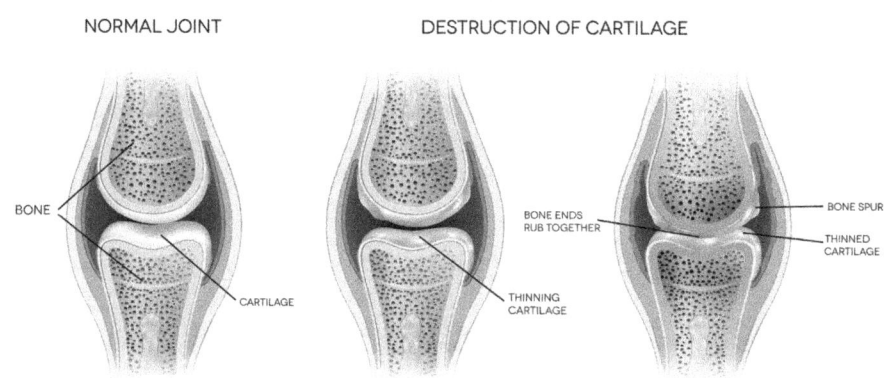

FIGURE 7-4: Osteoarthritis of the knee.

reineg/Adobe Stock Photos

Recognizing the signs of osteoarthritis

The signs and symptoms of osteoarthritis are the same in Western medicine and TCM, and each person who has arthritis experiences some combination of them in varying degrees:

» Pain or aching that's worse when you put weight on a joint (such as standing or carrying something heavy)

>> Stiffness after you're inactive for a long time (for example, after sleeping or sitting at work) that gets better after movement

>> Limited range of motion — your fingers, knees, or back don't straighten or bend fully

>> Cracking, grinding, or grating sensations (or sometimes sounds) when you move

>> Swelling around your joints

>> Joints that feel loose or unstable; for example, a knee that gives out from time to time

Identifying the arthritis problem

If you're a U.S. resident (or resident of any country that offers a Western medical system), you probably know the process of getting care through your primary care providers. It is similar in TCM, where the investigation of your problem starts when you report it to a TCM practitioner during a treatment session. As I detail in Chapter 6, your TCM practitioner draws on all their powers of deduction and the following senses:

>> **Talking:** Ask questions to get the full picture of what's happening in your body right now.

>> **Feeling:** Gently touch where you feel the pain, as well as feel your pulses on both wrists (see Chapter 6).

>> **Looking:** Observe the pain site(s) but also pay attention to your body language and facial expressions while you talk about your pain.

>> **Listening:** Actively listen to your answers and make sure that they hear and understand you correctly.

>> **Smelling:** Although not necessarily associated with pain, noticing smells can provide clues. For example, the scent of a topical pain reliever or marijuana can remind the practitioner to ask what you're already doing to manage your pain.

When you consult a TCM practitioner for any condition, they consider the internal and external influences that may be affecting you. In the case of osteoarthritis pain, they will consider Qi stagnation and the effect of environment pathogens, as I describe in the following sections.

Understanding the role of Qi stagnation

For all physical pain, the primary Qi problem is blocked Qi (in TCM terms, *Qi stagnation* or *Qi stasis*). The complicated part involves figuring out why the Qi isn't moving, where it got stuck, and which of the Five Elements categories, organ systems, and organ channels (or *meridians*) are involved.

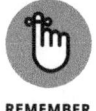

REMEMBER

In Chapter 2, I describe four basic *Qi* (energy) problems that form the basis of a TCM diagnosis:

>> Not enough Qi

>> Weak Qi

>> Blocked Qi

>> Wrong direction Qi

Discussed in more detail in Chapter 2, the Five Elements are Earth, Metal, Water, Wood, and Fire, which represent categories for organizing TCM concepts. The organ systems such as lungs, stomach, heart, and so on, are classified into one of these Five Elements categories, along with their corresponding organ channels (circulation pathways in the body).

Diagnosis and treatment are based on the Five Elements categories. So, in the case of pain, the practitioner determines which organ systems and channels are the source of the pain, as well as which organ systems and channels can be used to resolve the pain.

Considering environmental pathogens

TCM theory is the result of observations of humans and their interactions with the natural world. TCM commonly associates osteoarthritis with Qi that becomes stuck because of an environmental pathogen. *Environmental pathogens* are external influences that cause illness. Here are the environmental pathogens linked to osteoarthritis and joint pain and how they can affect you in the wider world:

>> **Wind:** Fighting against a strong wind that impedes your forward progress

>> **Damp:** Slogging through damp mud

>> **Cold:** Crunching on an ice cube

>> **Heat:** Lying motionless during a heat wave

These pathogens can affect people individually or in combination. All these natural elements can slow or halt movement, so the ancient practitioners witnessed and characterized osteoarthritis and joint pain in the body based on these elements.

Treating the arthritis problem with TCM

In simplest terms, TCM practitioners treat pain by achieving free flow of Qi in the body and the mind. Depending on the TCM diagnosis, all the TCM interventions can help treat almost any condition. In the following sections, I share the techniques that I find most effective in my practice for treating osteoarthritis and joint pain.

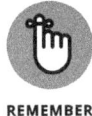

REMEMBER

The classic Traditional Chinese Medicine text *Huang Di Nei Jing* (which translates as *The Yellow Emperor's Classic of Medicine,* see Chapter 4 for more) states "if there is free flow, there is no pain; if there is no free flow, there is pain."

Using acupuncture for osteoarthritis pain

Like any blockage, the longer the Qi blockage goes unattended, the more solid it becomes and the harder it is for acupuncture treatment to clear it. *Auricular* (ear) acupuncture and other TCM therapies can reinforce acupuncture or replace it (if a patient has a fear of needles). Refer to Chapter 4 for more information on acupuncture.

Extensive research has shown that *acupuncture* (inserting sterile, hair-thin needles to stimulate specific points in the body) is highly effective as an *analgesic* (pain reliever), making it a viable alternative to powerful and highly addictive opioid painkillers such as morphine, codeine, oxycodone, hydrocodone, and fentanyl.

For arthritis and joint pain treatment, acupuncture practitioners typically select the acupuncture points (flip back to Chapter 4 for discussion of acupuncture points) located *locally* (near the site of pain) and *distally* (away from the pain site):

>> **Local points:** Applying acupuncture to these points breaks up the clog of Qi that causes the pain.

>> **Distal points:** Treating these acupuncture points flushes *Qi* (energy) along the organ channel(s).

TECHNICAL STUFF

The jury is out on how effective acupuncture is for osteoarthritis. Research on acupuncture specifically for osteoarthritis in various joints — from knees and elbows, to fingers and toes, to hips and shoulders — doesn't provide a consistent clear benefit. Despite this lack of consensus in research, some researchers consider acupuncture favorably as a supplement to conventional therapies, including medications such as nonsteroidal anti-inflammatory drugs (NSAIDs), such as Advil, or steroids, such as prednisone.

TIP

For patients who can't tolerate drugs, some research recommends acupuncture as an alternative. A *systematic review* (a comprehensive review of research on a specific topic that summarizes, assesses the validity of, and analyzes existing data) conducted in 2001 by the United Kingdom's National Health Service (NHS) — sort of a counterpart to Medicare/Medicaid in the U.S. — concluded that it had identified enough evidence to "justify the use of acupuncture as a second- or third-line treatment for a patient who's not responding to conventional management or not tolerating medication or experiencing recurrent pain."

Treating arthritis with tui na

A 2023 study published in the *Journal of Pain Research*, "Current Status of Research on Tuina for Analgesia," indicates that *tui na* (TCM therapeutic massage) has great potential as a nonpharmacological treatment for pain management based on the steadily increasing number of studies supporting tui na as an effective treatment for pain over the past 30 years.

These studies, such as a 2022 article in *Frontiers in Neuroscience* that reviewed the analgesic mechanism of tui na, show that tui na can effectively treat pain because it can release the blockage of *Qi* (energy) and blood along the organ channel(s). A practitioner can use tui na for all the joints and the supporting muscles, tendons, and tissue that surround the joints. Pressure, speed, duration, and technique (kneading, pushing, pulling, patting, pecking, and so on) vary depending on the diagnosis and the location of the joint pain. The practitioner feels for tender tissues, trigger points, contracted muscle tissue (called *knots*), and nodules to locate actual and referred pain sites. (*Referred pain sites* are areas where pain is felt, even though they're not the source of the pain.)

AUTHOR SAYS

Often, practitioners use tui na as a prelude to acupuncture (see the preceding section). Not many treatments use only tui na. I suspect that most patients don't know much about tui na and therefore expect to receive acupuncture as their primary therapy. Like any massage, tui na can be physically and energetically taxing. In a typical 50–60-minute session, I prefer to focus my efforts on the intake interview, diagnosis, and acupuncture treatment (see Chapter 6 for more on this process). Practitioners have the freedom to combine therapies as necessary to provide the relief and healing that individual patients need.

Creating arthritis treatments with herbal formulas

Taking aspirin is a one-size-fits-all remedy for pain. Practitioners customize TCM *herbal formulas* (recipes of herbal ingredients) designed to not only reduce pain but also target the underlying cause.

For a patient who has knee pain from a sports injury, for example, the practitioner selects herbs that move Qi and Blood (two vital substances in TCM theory), travel to the lower part of the body, and fortify the organ systems and organ channels associated with bones and tendons. See Chapter 2 to read more about TCM theory, including vital substances, organ systems, and channels. Acupuncture works from the outside in, while herbal formulas work from the inside out.

Of course, some herbal formulas are standardized: TCM has standard formulas that stand the test of millennia. And practitioners refined these formulas when they developed improved methods of growing, harvesting, and processing. Practitioners get the advantage of customizing a TCM herbal formula specifically for an individual patient. See Chapter 5 for more information on herbal formulas.

Heating arthritis pain with moxibustion

As described in Chapter 5, *moxibustion* delivers heat via the burning of mugwort indirectly over the surface of the skin or directly on the skin. Inserting a needle into the skin can transmit moxibustion heat beneath the surface of the skin. Heat expands and thereby can loosen tight muscles and strained tendons, and can dissolve knots and *adhesions* (bands of scar tissue). As TCM's equivalent to a heating pad or hot shower, moxibustion has a penetrating quality that opens the organ channels to restore the flow of energy for aching joints.

TECHNICAL
STUFF

In a 2022 article titled "The Case for Moxibustion for Painful Syndromes: History, principles and rationale," published in the *Current Research in Complementary & Alternative Medicine Journal,* the authors provide an overview of the use of moxibustion in China and Japan for thousands of years to maintain health and treat disease. The article also cites a variety of studies that show moxibustion to be an effective noninvasive therapy for pain reduction and management.

Another common form of arthritis is rheumatoid arthritis (RA). However, it's an autoimmune disease (where your immune system mistakenly attacks your body instead of defending it). Like osteoarthritis, RA causes pain, swelling, and stiffness in your joints. Unlike osteoarthritis, RA occurs in the same joints on both sides of your body and can lead to deformed joints. Because the causes of RA are so complex, I haven't addressed it here.

MAST CELLS: PROTECTORS OR PREDATORS?

When your immune system is functioning properly, it wards off illness and facilitates healing from injury. One of the key components of this system is mast cells, which patrol for things that can harm you like viruses, bacteria, parasites, toxins, and other substances. I was unaware of the importance of mast cells until my colleague Dr. DaGang Wang, DAOM, Dipl. O.M. (NCCAOM)®, L.Ac., called my attention to them.

When mast cells sense danger, they trigger your body's immune response to fight or remove the intruder. When mast cells are overzealous in their duties, you sneeze, itch, or have difficulty breathing because the mast cells are setting off a series of actions (too intricate to explain) to eliminate the offender. Food and environmental allergies, hives, and asthma are common examples of this, while anaphylaxis (severe, potentially life-threatening allergic reaction) is an extreme example of this.

Overactive mast cells can lead to chronic (long-term) inflammation like RA and also worsen other inflammatory disorders.

Lessening Back Pain

In 2017, the American College of Physicians (ACP) included acupuncture among the nondrug treatment options for the management of both acute and chronic low back pain as a result of evidence-based research.

LBP (*low back pain*; not *little black purse*) is so common that it has its own abbreviation. In fact, according to the American Association of Neurological Surgeons (AANS), an estimated 75–85 percent of people in the U.S. experience some kind of back pain in their lifetime.

TIP

In 2020, the Centers for Medicare and Medicaid Services (CMS) cited evidence reviews and the coverage policies of private payers for its decision to cover acupuncture for chronic low back pain. The addition of acupuncture to CMS coverage opened the door for other insurance providers to include acupuncture as a covered service.

If you have Medicare or Medicaid coverage, you can ask your TCM practitioner if they accept it. If you don't have this coverage, this is an opportunity to ask your insurance provider to cover acupuncture because CMS does.

For more information on CMS coverage of acupuncture, please visit https://www.medicare.gov/coverage/acupuncture. The site also offers a provider search at https://www.medicare.gov/care-compare/.

Recognizing the signs of back pain

People often experience back pain because of muscle strain from lifting, exercising, falling, or being in an accident. Other causes include nerve compression (also known as a *pinched nerve*), osteoarthritis, and *spinal stenosis* (narrowing of the spinal cord pathway). (Back pain can also be a symptom of more complex issues, such as pregnancy or cancer, which I discuss in Chapter 10.)

The signs and symptoms of back pain are the same in Western medicine and TCM, and each person experiences some combination of them in varying degrees:

>> Pain worsens with movement and improves with rest

>> Pain with coughing or sneezing (if you have nerve compression)

>> Limited range of motion — you can't turn, bend, or straighten your back

The actual pain sensation depends on the cause:

>> **Tight and achy:** Muscle strain

>> **Sharp or throbbing or intermittently numb:** Nerve compression/stenosis

>> **All of the above:** Osteoarthritis

Identifying the causes of back pain

The same process of inquiry goes into assessing back pain as for arthritis and joint pain (which I talk about in the section "Reducing Arthritis and Joint Pain," earlier in this chapter), and TCM attributes back pain to the same Qi problems and environmental pathogens. (Spinal arthritis presents as low back and/or neck pain.) However, back pain can be a symptom of a wide range of conditions, such as obesity, diabetes, gout, irritable bowel syndrome (IBS), and Lyme disease. Structural problems, such as *scoliosis* (a condition where the spine curves like an S), can further complicate the investigation into the causes of back pain.

The basic Qi problem remains the same: Blocked Qi. However, the underlying cause can involve a combination of all four Qi problems outlined in Chapter 2. In the case of spinal arthritis, the same environmental pathogens as arthritis and joint pain may be in play, but back pain caused by other conditions requires much more intricate evaluation and diagnosis.

Working the back-pain problem with TCM

A practitioner can use any and all of the therapies that I describe for arthritis and joint pain in the section "Reducing Arthritis and Joint Pain," earlier in this chapter, to treat back pain, so I describe modifications for those therapies in the following sections. I also discuss an additional treatment for back pain — cupping — in the section "Cupping to treat back pain," later in this chapter.

Treating back pain with acupuncture

A 2017 study published in *Medical Acupuncture* ("Reduction in Pain Medication Prescriptions and Self-Reported Outcomes Associated with Acupuncture in a Military Patient Population") examined using acupuncture to help reduce reliance on medication in the military. The study included 172 patients who received a minimum of four acupuncture treatments over the course of one year at the Mike O'Callaghan Military Medical Center at Nellis Air Force Base in Nevada. The study reported that "opioid prescriptions decreased by 45 percent, muscle relaxants by 34 percent, NSAIDs by 42 percent, and benzodiazepines by 14 percent."

Depending on the underlying cause(s) of the back pain, the TCM practitioner targets acupuncture points on the back, as well as points related to the primary organ systems and organ channels (see Chapter 2) involved in the underlying cause(s). In chronic cases that involve *comorbidities* (unrelated medical conditions), releasing the blockage may take some time.

Cupping to treat back pain

Cupping, using glass or plastic cups to stimulate muscle tissue (see Chapter 5), is particularly effective in large areas of the body, such as the back, because it improves blood and lymph circulation.

Cups vary in size, and each size has a different degree of suction. The suction from the cups enhances circulation and releases tension. The practitioner can leave the cups stationary for a more intense effect or can move them over the body's surface for more coverage and less intensity, depending on the practitioner's technique.

TECHNICAL STUFF

In 2024, *Complementary Therapies in Medicine* published a systematic review of 11 studies that assessed the effectiveness of cupping therapy on low back pain. Based on their analysis, the review determined that high- and moderate-quality evidence indicated that cupping significantly improved pain and disability. The effectiveness of cupping varied according to duration of treatment, type of cupping technique, and type of back pain. The review stated, "Cupping demonstrated a superior and sustained effect on pain reduction compared with medication and usual care."

Using herbal formulas to treat back pain

As noted in the section "Creating arthritis treatments with herbal formulas," earlier in this chapter, extensive research has been conducted on individual herbs from the TCM *materia medica* (plant, animal, and mineral products used medically).

Although I can't discuss every herb that can help alleviate pain in this book, one that has been studied extensively is Corydalis Rhizoma (*yan hu suo*). This herb's active ingredients appear to block or mute pain signals, relax muscles and blood vessels, and activate *dopamine* (the feel-good hormone). It also impedes the release of *histamine* (a chemical that has a primary role in the body's immune and allergic response) and *pro-inflammatory mediators* (molecules and proteins that facilitate the body's inflammatory response). In TCM language, Corydalis Rhizoma is a powerful mover of Qi and Blood, which makes it ideal for unblocking Qi (see Chapter 2). Figure 7-5 shows cut-and-dried Corydalis rhizomes that have become yan hu suo.

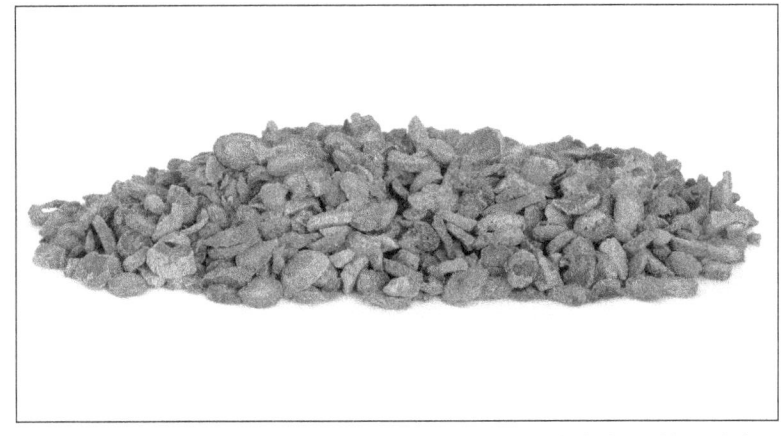

FIGURE 7-5: Corydalis rhizomes that have been dried and cut to become yan hu suo.

marilyn barbone/Adobe Stock Photos

For a patient who has back pain, the practitioner selects herbs such as Corydalis Rhizoma that move Qi and Blood and combines them with others that travel to the back of the body and fortify the organ systems and organ channels associated with the spine. The practitioner also uses additional herbs to address any underlying causes that contribute to the patient's back pain.

TECHNICAL STUFF

To read about studies that show how well single herbs, compounds, or extracts of TCM work for pain management, check out *Advances in Pharmacology* (Elsevier, Inc.), published in 2016 (Volume 75).

Alleviating Headache

Headaches are pain anywhere on the head, including the scalp, upper neck, face, and interior of the skull. Headaches can be a fleeting nuisance or debilitating. Some people have them frequently, while others rarely do. Headaches have two types of causes:

>> **Primary:** Originating in the head area

>> **Secondary:** Caused by another condition, outside of the head

In the following sections, I focus on primary headaches, which include tension headaches (the most common of all headaches) and migraines.

Recognizing the signs of a headache

Tension headaches come from experiencing events in everyday life, such as stress, lack of sleep, or staring at a computer screen, TV, or phone for too long. In addition to the causes of tension headaches, a host of other factors, such as changing weather conditions, fluctuating hormones, and overstimulation from lights or smells, can trigger migraines. Tension headaches are rarely severe and don't often put you out of commission. In comparison (and confirmed by anyone who's had one), there's no such thing as a mild migraine.

AUTHOR SAYS

Although researchers haven't clearly identified why, studies show that more women than men have tension headaches, and migraines affect women three times more than men. While my patient population is a small sample, this is pretty accurate. I rarely see men with headaches, and I see women who suffer from tension headaches and migraines regularly.

The signs and symptoms of headaches are the same in Western medicine and TCM. Table 7-1 can help you distinguish between tension headaches and migraines.

TABLE 7-1   **Primary Headaches**

Characteristics	Episodic Tension Headaches	Chronic Tension Headaches	Migraine Headaches
Frequency	Fewer than 15 days per month	More than 15 days per month	Usually episodic
Pain level	Mild to moderate	Varies in intensity	Moderate to severe
Duration	30 minutes to several days; starts after waking and gets worse throughout the day	Remains constant for more than 15 days/month	Four hours to several days
Sensation	A tight band around the head, starting at the front or the eyes, and then spreading over the rest of the head	A tight band around the head, starting at the front or the eyes, and then spreading over the rest of the head	Pulsing or throbbing Accompanied by nausea and sensitivity to light, sound, and/or smell
Onset age	Teens	Teens	Puberty or young adulthood

Identifying the problem causing headaches

Each of the 12 major channels, plus the Du and Ren extra channels, is connected to the head (see Chapter 2). So, in addition to the blocked *Qi* (energy) problem, a patient who experiences headaches probably has either:

» **Weak Qi:** Can't ward off the effects of wind, cold, heat, or damp (see "Identifying the arthritis problem" earlier in this chapter)

» **Not enough Qi and/or Blood:** In one or more channels; doesn't provide the head with balanced sustenance

So, how does a practitioner sift through the evidence from all these different channels? Location, location, location. One of the biggest clues in addressing headaches in TCM is where the pain occurs:

» **Pain in the back of the neck with a backache:** Small Intestine and Urinary Bladder

» **Pain across the forehead and/or radiating down to the top of the eye socket:** Large Intestine and Stomach

» **Pain on both sides of the head, more intense at the temples:** San Jiao and Gallbladder

» **Pain with a sensation of heaviness in the head, plus abdominal bloating and spontaneous sweating:** Lung and Spleen

>> **Pain that radiates in the skull and teeth:** Heart and Kidney

>> **Pain at the top and corners of the head, a sensation of air rising like a balloon in the head, and nausea/vomiting:** Pericardium and Liver

The location of the headache, combined with other signs and symptoms, and examination of your tongue and pulse (see Chapter 6) allow the practitioner to choose the acupuncture points appropriately.

Working the headache problem with TCM

The following therapies can treat headaches. Like with all things TCM, the choice of therapy depends on the individual patient and the practitioner's diagnosis.

Practicing acupuncture for headaches

It may seem counterintuitive to insert needles in a headache sufferer's head. But a combination of acupuncture on the body, scalp, and ears can provide significant and sustained relief. In some cases, using *electrostimulation* (administering a low-frequency electrical current through the needles) may reduce the dilation (widening) of blood vessels that contribute to migraine.

Based on pain location and other signs and symptoms, the practitioner selects the appropriate acupuncture points to use, as well as any supplemental therapy.

One of acupuncture's limitations is that it's not a one-and-done treatment. For those suffering from chronic headaches, treatment at consistent intervals for a sustained timeframe is most effective. On the other hand, acupuncture's advantages may outweigh this limitation. It's convenient, safe, nonaddictive, and long-lasting when the patient receives consistent treatment.

TECHNICAL STUFF

An exhaustive review of research literature on acupuncture and migraine, "Efficacy of Acupuncture-Related Therapy for Migraine: A Systematic Review and Network Meta-Analysis," was published in 2024 in the *Journal of Pain Research.* More than 1,800 articles and 34 studies were included in the assessment, and the reviewers determined that acupuncture was more effective than medication in reducing the severity, frequency, and duration of migraine attacks.

Treating headaches with herbal formulas

I like to think of herbs as the treatment that you take with you. In the section "Using herbal formulas to treat back pain," earlier in this chapter, I mentioned Corydalis Rhizoma. Herbal formulas often pair it with another well-studied herb,

Radix Angelica dahurica (*Bai Zhi*), another root that also has *analgesic* (pain relieving) and anti-inflammatory properties, but it works on different chemicals and pathways in the body.

Although Corydalis Rhizoma can effectively treat many types of pain, Radix Angelica dahurica specifically helps treat *vertex* (top of the head), sinus, *orbital* (behind the eyes), and virus-related (cold or flu) headaches. With these two herbs taking the lead, additional herbs can serve as the backup to support their actions or to offset properties of these pain-relieving herbs that the patient doesn't need.

Using tui na to treat headaches

Through its manipulation of soft tissue, tui na appears to activate or release chemical molecules that affect sensory nerve endings. All massage likely has this effect; however, tui na works the organ channels to help loosen blocked *Qi* (energy). A practitioner might use tui na as the warm-up act before the headliner treatment or as the final act of a drama where the story gets resolved.

Research on tui na specifically for headaches is limited. *Complementary Therapies in Clinical Practice* in 2021 published a systematic review of seven studies involving tui na for tension headaches, "The effectiveness and safety of Tuina for tension-type headache: A systematic review and meta-analysis." Although it didn't come to any definitive conclusions (research papers rarely do), the review determined that tui na reduced the VAS score (see below) for tension headaches.

The Visual Analog Scale (VAS) measures pain intensity by having patients report their level of pain on a 10-point scale. See Figure 7-6.

VISUAL ANALOG SCALE

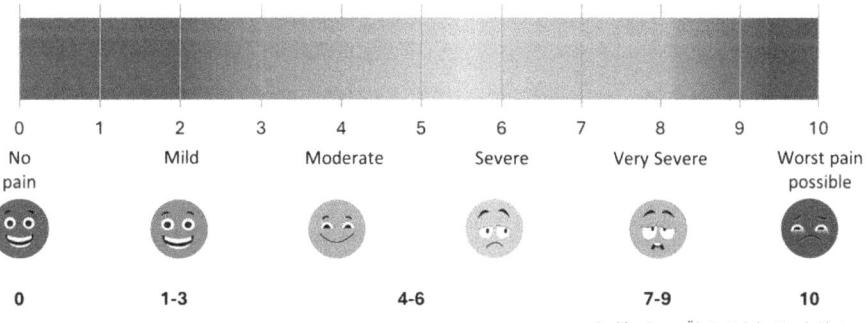

FIGURE 7-6:
The Visual Analog Scale (VAS) is commonly used for patients to report their level of pain.

Bediha Duru Öksüz/Adobe Stock Photos

Treating headaches with cupping

The most recent research I could find on cupping was a review of cupping for migraine published in 2021. It was found that cupping was beneficial for migraine treatment, but they couldn't downright confirm it.

The review recommended further study because cupping had the potential to effectively treat headaches, mainly because it has similar effects on the nervous system as tui na (see the preceding section). I don't have a sample size in my clinical practice large enough to qualify as research, but two-thirds of my patients who receive cupping regularly tend to fall asleep during the therapy. I interpret this reaction as turning down the volume on pain and tuning out.

Chapter **8**

Managing Addictions and Mental Health

This chapter deals with difficult health conditions that many people don't feel comfortable discussing. The common denominators in all of them involve behaviors and the brain.

Although people find all serious health problems challenging and distressing, many of the conditions in this chapter can lay waste to not only a person's health but also their relationships, finances, and sense of self. I know because I've experienced this as someone who has suffered recurrent depressive episodes since my early 30s. Traditional Chinese Medicine (TCM) can help people experiencing issues in these areas, and I'm grateful for the opportunity to share how.

Considering How TCM Views Mental Health

In Chapter 2, I introduce concepts that are fundamental to TCM theory. Most of those concepts relate to the physical aspects of health because these aspects are what most of us deal with daily — aches, pains, indigestion, the common cold, tiredness, and so on. Also, I've tried to stick to the fundamentals like the student I was when I began my TCM education.

Oddly, the textbook that is one of the primary resources for examination and licensure (see Chapter 3) in California and widely used internationally as a standard reference — *Chinese Acupuncture and Moxibustion* (Foreign Languages Press) — says very little about mental health. Aside from six paragraphs on the emotions associated with the organs (see Chapter 2) and a discussion of the brain as an extra organ responsible for thinking, manic-depressive disorder (or *bipolar disorder*) is the only mental health condition cited in the entire book. Consequently, the curriculum at my school was limited in formal education on this topic.

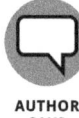

AUTHOR SAYS

I don't think the textbook authors or my alma mater meant to leave out what I believe is the most critical half of the mind–body connection; the half that moves our bodies, wills us to live, motivates our choices, and makes each of us a unique thinking and feeling human. It may have been too daunting, too delicate, and too intricate to translate the information, let alone try to explain it.

This chapter is an attempt to offer you a small window into the mind from a TCM perspective by distilling everything I've learned since 2010 from my professors, clinic supervisors, elective courses, continuing education courses, books, patients, and personal struggles.

Defining the Spirit

In TCM, the mental, emotional, and spiritual workings of a human being are represented by the Chinese word *Shen*, which is typically translated as *Spirit*. I consider *Shen* to be the equivalent of *psyche*, which is defined by the American Psychological Association as "the mind in its totality, as distinguished from the physical organism," and comes from the Greek word for soul — *psychē*.

To incorporate the nonphysical aspects of human life into their understanding of illness and health, the ancient physicians and scholars conceived of the Spirit as a combination of five essential sub-spirits that are individual but inseparable. These five spirits are associated with the five *Zang* organs (see Chapter 2): Heart, Spleen, Lung, Kidney, and Liver.

> **» Shen (Heart):** Yes, it's the same word, but as a sub-spirit, this *shen* is associated with connection, communication, propriety, and relating to others and the world rationally.
>
> During my depressive episodes, I withdrew from my family and friends, and I refused to leave the house. I had difficulty expressing myself, and I spoke

slowly, if I spoke at all. This behavior is not uncommon for others who also experience depression.

» **Yi (Spleen):** This sub-spirit is the decision-maker, planner, and evaluator of choices and possibilities. It can be translated as intention or consciousness, but it also involves insight and intuition. This is thinking that directs action and delivers a result.

The worst aspect of my depressive episodes was my inability to decide anything. I couldn't choose what to wear or what to eat. Getting out of bed presented the challenge of what to do next, which would then spiral into fretting about doing nothing. For some people with depression, this can manifest as confusion or laziness.

» **Po (Lung):** This sub-spirit is translated as *animal soul* or *corporeal soul.* This sub-spirit is responsible for feelings and emotions in the moment. It includes spontaneity, reactivity, responsiveness, and decisiveness.

When I was depressed, I was Winnie-the-Pooh's Eeyore in the flesh. Like others who experience depressive episodes, what looked like disinterest to my friends and family was me shutting down.

» **Zhi (Kidney):** This sub-spirit is translated as *will,* and it is the drive, determination, and persistence that reaches goals. It also involves consistency, reliability, and steadiness.

In my depressed state, I wanted to abandon the life and career I had established and move back in with my parents, so they could drive while I sat in the back seat. For those experiencing a depressive episode, taking the path of least resistance seems like a good choice.

» **Hun (Liver):** This sub-spirit can be difficult to understand. The word most commonly used in reference to *hun* is *soul*.

In *The Foundations of Chinese Medicine,* Giovanni Maciocia writes, "The Ethereal Soul is responsible for our life's dreams, plans, ideas, projects, sense of purpose, relationship with other people, etc."

In *The Web That Has No Weaver,* Ted J. Kaptchuk, O.M.D., states, "An intact *Hun* produces acts of kindness or benevolence toward others and self. If the *Hun* is not intact, a person can be unkind toward others (e.g., overly angry and belligerent) or unkind to himself or herself (e.g., unable to feel self-worth or be self-deprecating)."

Taken together, I interpret *hun* to be the spirit that gives me a reason for being. Also, it fosters empathy, compassion, and humanity. During my worst depressive episode, I felt unworthy of the love and concern of my family and friends, and I lost my reason for being. To me, this is the deepest level of depression for people — when they lose purpose and passion.

Treating the Spirit(s)

At a very basic level, TCM practitioners treat the Spirit (and its sub-spirits) when they treat mental and behavioral health conditions. Some of these conditions can originate from a physical illness like chronic pain. Some can originate from a traumatic or shocking event like a war, a natural disaster, a crime, or an unexpected loss of a loved one.

Like physical health issues, some mental and behavioral health issues, such as autism, can be genetic or inherited. Of course, just because you have relatives with a genetic or inherited condition doesn't mean you will develop that condition; it just means you might be more likely to develop it than someone without the condition in their family medical history. Some mental and behavioral health issues, such as post-traumatic stress disorder, crop up immediately after a crisis or trauma. Other mental and behavioral health issues build over time or result from an accumulation of stressors, such as was the case with my own depressive episodes, which I'll share more in sections on common disorders and TCM treatments later in this chapter.

The trick, as with every health condition, is to figure out where and how the condition started, and how to provide patients with relief from their suffering.

Defining Addiction and Mental Health

The stigma that many cultures place around addiction and mental health conditions makes it difficult for people to acknowledge when they need help. Although making it an identifiable problem may ease the perception, you can't allow familiarity to reduce the seriousness or severity of the issue.

Referring to addictions and mental health issues as "problems" may seem too simplistic, but it's the most common term I hear when people discuss these conditions. For example:

>> They have a problem with alcohol.

>> They have a problem with food.

>> Schools offer interventions like social skills training and counseling to deal with behavioral problems.

>> This generation has a lot of substance abuse problems.

Identifying the problem

Addiction and mental health conditions can be life-threatening. Preliminary data from the Centers for Disease Control and Prevention (CDC) show that suicide claimed more than 49,000 people in 2023, and the National Center for Health Statistics (a unit of the CDC) provides data that indicates state and local health jurisdictions reported 80,674 drug overdose deaths in the U.S. between November 2023 and November 2024.

I can't change the way anyone talks about addiction or mental health, but I do think you need to use accurate terminology so that you and your health-care providers are on the same page.

Addiction

The American Society of Addiction Medicine (ASAM) characterizes *addiction* as a treatable disease that involves brain chemistry, genetics, environmental factors, and a person's lived experience. Even though addiction is harmful, those suffering from it are unable to control their intense need for a substance like alcohol or their impulse to excessively engage in a certain behavior like eating or gambling.

Addictions fall into two main categories:

» Substance use disorders (SUDs), such as:

- Alcohol
- Caffeine
- Opioids (such as oxycodone and heroin)
- Sedatives (typically used for sleep or relaxation)
- Stimulants (including cocaine)
- Tobacco/nicotine (smoking)

» Non-substance/behavioral addictions:

- Behaviors related to food, such as not eating or overeating
- Gambling
- Shoplifting or other risky behaviors
- Shopping
- Video gaming (internet gaming disorder; IGD)
- Behaviors related to sex, such as watching pornography or engaging with multiple partners

AUTHOR
SAYS

Behavioral addictions like those listed above are much more complicated than a substance addiction because it's very difficult to avoid eating, shopping, or having sex. As someone who has organized a March Madness pool for the national college basketball tournament for decades, even a little gambling comes into play on the regular. In TCM, uncovering the root cause(s) of a behavioral addiction and treating it involves more knowledge than I have to convey. In my own clinical experience, I have reduced the level of craving for a short period of time, but I haven't contributed to a sustained change in behavior. Therefore, I've only addressed SUDs here.

According to the 2023 United States National Survey on Drug Use and Health, 48.5 million (16.7 percent) of Americans aged 12 and older battled an SUD in the previous 12 months.

Statistics vary on the different behavioral addictions because researchers don't agree on the criteria for diagnosis. For example, the National Council on Problem Gambling cites that 2.5 million (1 percent) U.S. adults meet the criteria for a severe gambling disorder; while 5 to 8 million (2–3 percent) meet some of them, and therefore, face life difficulties (which the study didn't detail) because of gambling. Estimates for video game addiction range from 1.7 to 10 percent of the U.S. population.

TECHNICAL
STUFF

Organizations that research and track health care statistics globally and nationally consider the U.S. among the most addicted countries in the world. From drugs to tobacco to screen time, data from multiple sources like the CDC, United Nations, World Health Organization, and the Commonwealth Fund seem to support this conclusion. For a deeper dive into global drug use statistics, you can check out `https://ourworldindata.org/illicit-drug-use`.

Mental health

The Substance Abuse and Mental Health Services Administration (SAMHSA) website states that *mental health*:

> . . .includes our emotional, psychological, and social well-being. It affects how we think, feel, and act, and helps determine how we handle stress, relate to others, and make choices.

Many of the factors involved in addiction are also involved in mental health disorders — genes, brain chemistry, life experience, and family history. Mental health disorders include:

>> Anxiety, including generalized anxiety, panic disorders, obsessive-compulsive disorder (OCD), phobias, and social anxiety

- » Attention-deficit hyperactivity disorder (ADHD)
- » Depression
- » Eating disorders, including anorexia nervosa, binge eating disorder, and bulimia nervosa
- » Post-traumatic stress disorder (PTSD)

SAMHSA notes that almost one out of five people (20 percent) in the U.S. live with a mental health disorder. The 2023 United States National Survey on Drug Use and Health reported that 20.4 million American adults (7.9 percent) suffered from both a mental health disorder and an SUD — double trouble.

Finding help

The United States has a plethora of resources and national organizations to help people with the addictions or mental health issues. Flip to Appendix A for a list of some of them.

Many mental health conditions are preventable or treatable. Data varies, but some estimates say that only 8–14 percent of those with 12-month SUDs sought treatment or help. An estimated 50 percent of those who have mental health disorders seek treatment or help. As someone who asked for help, I wouldn't be here without the support of my family and friends and the treatment that I received.

I experienced three depressive episodes before I discovered TCM and one afterward. So, TCM can't serve as a magic wand that whisks away the trouble or keeps it from coming back. For me, it was the life raft that kept me from drowning before a comprehensive treatment plan combining TCM with an antidepressant and psychotherapy could take hold.

Curbing Uncontrolled Cravings

Public awareness campaigns, medical research, and drug development have long focused on substance use disorders (SUDs). But these addictions remain the source of several chronic diseases and premature death, and a huge amount of medical and financial resources go to treating them.

The societal costs of substance abuse vary depending on what exactly the researchers measure and how they collect the data. One investigation published in 2022 on JAMA (*Journal of the American Medical Association*) evaluated the cost of

SUDs among workers who had employer insurance. Out of 162 million insured workers, 2.3 million (1.4 percent) had a substance use disorder (SUD) diagnosis in 2018. The total annual cost for just medical services for this group was $35.3 billion! Alcohol use disorder cost $10.2 billion, and opioid use disorder cost $7.3 billion.

Because I associate addiction with *uncontrolled craving* — wanting or needing something so intensely you'll do anything to get it, regardless of the consequences — the following sections explore the treatment options for SUDs only.

Using the NADA protocol

No one plans to develop an SUD. As a very simple explanation, these substances can make you feel good. They calm you, take away pain, elevate your mood, "drown your sorrows," and so on.

TCM practitioners have only recently started using TCM therapies to treat addiction, compared to its long history (and by long, I mean thousands of years) as a therapy to maintain health and treat illness.

The discovery of how acupuncture can help treat addictions happened by fortunate accident. In 1972, Hsiang-Lai Wen, a Hong Kong neurosurgeon, was treating a 50-year-old man who had a concussion. The patient also happened to be an opium addict who suffered withdrawal symptoms while in the hospital. He received an opium tincture to ease his suffering and also received electroacupuncture (which I talk about in Chapter 4) for pain relief (see Chapter 7 for discussion of headaches). Lo and behold, the patient reported not only being relieved of pain but also relieved of his withdrawal symptoms. The next time he suffered from withdrawal, they used electroacupuncture again, and his symptoms subsided.

After this unexpected turn of events, Wen and his colleague Dr. S.Y.C. Cheung tried to achieve similar results with 40 other patients. They published their findings in an article in the *Asian Journal of Medicine* in 1973 that demonstrated the efficacy of acupuncture for heroin and opium withdrawal symptoms and established a treatment protocol. The protocol involved inserting acupuncture needles into both ears and then stimulating the needles with a low-level electric current. News of their promising discovery was shared in a *New York Times* article, published on April 5, 1973, "Hong Kong Doctors Use Acupuncture to Relieve Addicts' Withdrawal Symptoms."

Located in the South Bronx, New York, Lincoln Hospital created one of the first detoxification programs in the U.S. for heroin addicts in 1970, spurred by the activism of a coalition of civil rights groups, including the Young Lords, Black Panthers, and their allies. With community and hospital support, as well as the cooperation of the City, the coalition and staff and community volunteers transformed the hospital auditorium into a drug detox clinic. Initially, patients received decreasing doses of methadone to be detoxed. But rather than trading one drug for another, they sought nonpharmaceutical interventions. After learning about Wen's findings, they adopted his acupuncture protocol at the clinic. Through clinical use and observation, practitioners simplified the protocol to five *auriculotherapy* (needling on the ear; see Chapter 4 for more on this technique) points without the use of electrical stimulation, as shown in Figure 8-1.

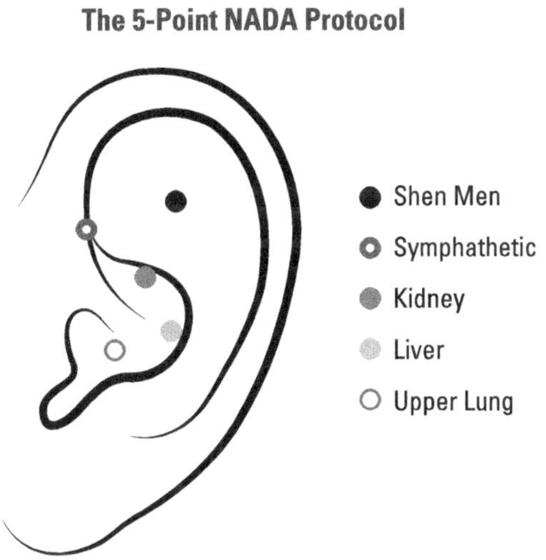

The 5-Point NADA Protocol

- ● Shen Men
- ◉ Symphathetic
- ◔ Kidney
- ◌ Liver
- ○ Upper Lung

FIGURE 8-1: The 5-point NADA protocol.

Other clinical practitioners in the U.S. and other countries soon adopted the protocol. Unfortunately, Lincoln Detox was closed by then-Mayor Edward Koch in 1978. However, some Lincoln members founded another program nearby, called the Lincoln Recovery Center, and in 1985, the Center's Director, Michael O. Smith, M.D., D.Ac., founded the National Acupuncture Detoxification Association (NADA). Dr. Smith (who passed away in 2017) was an associate professor of psychiatry at Cornell Medical School, an acupuncturist, and a noted addiction specialist. Through his leadership, NADA codified the protocol, which now goes by the name the NADA protocol (for obvious reasons). NADA trains acupuncture detoxification specialists (ADSs) who receive combined classroom and hands-on practical instruction throughout the U.S. and 17 other countries.

The NADA protocol offers some advantages over standard addiction treatments, such as medications like methadone for opioids and naltrexone for alcohol. Medication therapy is commonly combined with behavioral counseling. A practitioner can use the NADA protocol anywhere, and it's safe for children, teens, and pregnant women.

Also, by using the NADA protocol, you don't have to worry about:

>> Side effects (unless the practitioner doesn't correctly follow the Clean Needle Technique; see Chapter 6)

>> A practitioner's need for years of additional training and tuition

>> Needles; the practitioner can use *ear seeds* (tiny acacia seeds affixed to the ear with adhesive) or magnetic beads instead

Depending on U.S. state laws and approval, a variety of professionals can become certified as an ADS, including:

>> Addiction and harm reduction counselors

>> Mental health therapists and social workers

>> Correctional officers and drug court personnel

>> Disaster relief teams and trauma support center staff

>> First responders, nurses, and EMTs

>> Acupuncturists and medical doctors

The NADA protocol also doesn't cost a lot, in terms of time or money:

>> Treatment times can last between 35 and 45 minutes.

>> Practitioners can treat patients in groups, requiring fewer personnel (one practitioner can treat multiple patients) and less equipment and facilities (needles, chairs, a room or two); a savings they hopefully pass on to their patients.

TCM's NADA protocol can treat a variety of addictions, including:

>> Opioids, cocaine, and heroin

>> Alcohol

>> Nicotine (the addictive chemical in tobacco)

>> Gambling

Auriculotherapy can help relieve withdrawal symptoms, reduce the rate of treatment dropouts, and curb cravings.

Cutting down on smoking

According to the CDC, smoking appeals to the chemical receptors of nearly one out of five — about 49.2 million — U.S. adults. The data doesn't count the kids in middle school and high school who favor e-cigarettes and nicotine pouches that replicate smoking tobacco, according to the American Lung Association. The 2024 National Youth Tobacco Survey reported that 10.1 percent of high school students and 5.4 percent of middle school students use at least one tobacco product.

In terms of costs, smoking causes the deaths of over 490,000 people a year, and secondhand smoke causes over 19,000 deaths a year. As the number one preventable cause of death, smoking costs over $600 billion in direct healthcare costs and lost productivity annually.

Because nicotine is a highly addictive substance, people who smoke fall into the category of folks who have an SUD; they can receive treatment accordingly, with standard interventions such as psychotherapy and medications (for example, patches or nasal sprays that replace nicotine).

Typical TCM approaches to encouraging smoking cessation include acupuncture with or without electric current, *acupressure* (hand or finger pressure), and herbal medicine. The NADA protocol (discussed in the preceding section) provides an effective therapy for smoking cessation.

Easing the Mind

As I note at the beginning of this chapter, one of the primary texts for my education and licensing, *Chinese Acupuncture and Moxibustion (CAM),* doesn't contain much information about psychology or mental health disorders. However, in describing the functions and responsibilities of the *zang* organs (see Chapter 2), there is a short discussion of the *mind.* According to CAM, "the word 'mind' has the broad meaning of the . . . . vital activities of the whole body, and the narrow meaning of consciousness, e.g., spirit and thinking." One of the functions of the *Heart* is to house the *mind,* as described in the foundational ancient text, *The Emperor's Yellow Canon* (see Chapter 4).

Earlier in this chapter, I also introduced you to the concepts of the Spirit (*Shen*) and its smaller sub-spirits (*shen, yi, po, zhi,* and *hun*) with their organ associations. Given the mind's affiliation with the *Heart* and the sub-spirits' affiliations with the five *zang* (heart, spleen, lung, kidney, and liver), mental health in TCM is closely linked to the balanced functioning of the body, and physical health is closely linked to the harmonious functioning of the mind.

REMEMBER

When developing TCM theory, the ancient physicians didn't have the advantage of modern technology or techniques to gain a full understanding of the brain. Yet, they did consider the brain to be overrated as the "nucleus" of the body. Instead, the ancient physicians truly embraced the concept of the "body-mind," understanding that consciousness exists in all our organs, as well as within our blood.

The American Psychiatric Association (APA) considers TCM to be:

> "an excellent complementary alternative to contemporary treatments for physical and mental health needs. Integrating TCM with modern healthcare enriches the available treatment options and aligns with the shift towards a more holistic and integrated approach to care; this cultural blend enhances the healing process, combining time-tested methods with current medical advancements."

I can't say it any better. Earlier in this chapter, I listed a handful of mental and behavioral health conditions that afflict millions of people. In this section, I discuss three conditions that are widespread, that I have encountered in my patients, and that I have experienced personally.

Managing stress

Stress — everyone experiences it at some time or another, and each of us responds to and copes with it in our own way. It can come at you from different *stressors* (sources of stress) in minor, major, and overwhelming ways — broken dishwasher; traffic; issues with work, school, family, or friends; violence and abuse situations; a natural disaster; and so on.

The body's response to stressors

TECHNICAL STUFF

The healthcare profession widely recognizes that stress is the precursor to many diseases, both physical and mental. The concept of maintaining a stable internal environment was described by French physiologist Claude Bernard in 1849 and was named *homeostasis* by Harvard physiologist Walter Bradford Cannon in 1926. In 1956, Austrian-born Canadian endocrinologist Hans Selye theorized that any serious threat to homeostasis was a *stressor* and the body's reaction to that stressor was the *stress response*. Known as the father of stress research, Selye surmised that intense, long-term stress responses cause tissue damage and disease.

The stress response, or more commonly known as the *fight or flight response*, signals your body to face a threat or run from it — your heart pumps harder and faster, your muscles tense, your breath quickens, your brain activity increases;

even your immune system activates. After you recognize that the threat has passed, your body returns to normal function. But if your body and brain remain on high alert, the physical and mental response can disrupt almost all your functions. This continuous stress state puts you at increased risk for a range of health issues, from pain and allergies to sleep and mental health disorders, to cardiovascular disease and diabetes, to autoimmune disorders.

Therapies for stress reduction

Fortunately, your body and brain can adapt and heal, and you can manage and modify your stress response. You can figure out how to identify what stresses you and how to take care of yourself. In other words, you can become more resilient.

Because TCM therapies focus on the prevention of physical ailments, they can effectively support resilience. TCM therapies can help you heal and recover from any number of life's stressors:

» **Acupuncture:** Researchers associate the effect of acupuncture with regulating *dopamine* (the "feel-good" hormone or "reward and motivation" hormone; see Appendix B) and decreasing *cortisol* (the stress hormone). In particular, electroacupuncture can create *hemodynamic* (cardiovascular function) changes in a wide range of brain networks, which can have therapeutic effects on a variety of areas, including emotion, sensation, movement, and pain reduction.

» **Qigong:** This breath and movement therapy can promote relaxation and reduce stress by quieting the mind and regulating the nervous system. When you combine Qigong movements, as shown in Figure 8-2, with deep breathing techniques, you can help release tension and promote a sense of calmness. Research has shown that regular Qigong practice can reduce feelings of anxiety, depression, and mood swings.

» **Traditional Chinese Herbs (TCH):** Although researchers haven't done a lot of studies on the effect of TCH on stress specifically, TCM employs a range of herbal formulas tailored to individuals to help improve mood, reduce the stress response, and enhance overall mental well-being. Because, in TCM theory, most mental and emotional stressors relate to imbalances in the Liver and Heart channels (and their associated sub-spirits, *hun* and *shen*, respectively), a TCM practitioner creates a specific formula that addresses the imbalance in the Liver and/or Heart functions to improve depression or ease the stress response.

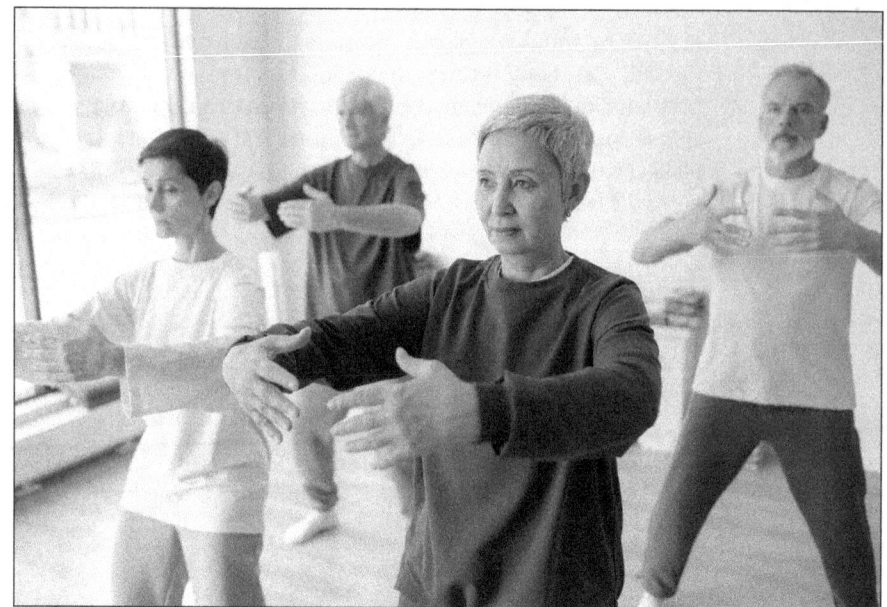

FIGURE 8-2:
Qigong practice is
known to be
physically,
mentally, and
spiritually
rehabilitative.

Seventyfour/Adobe Stock Photos

Overcoming trauma

Although healthcare professionals widely recognize and use acupuncture to treat physical or neurological pain, research suggests that it also offers benefits in the treatment of mental pain from trauma.

The organization Acupuncturists Without Borders (AWB), founded in 2005 and modeled along the lines of Doctors Without Borders, provides acupuncture in disaster-impacted communities. In a 2023 guest editorial in the journal *Medical Acupuncture*, Program Director Carla Cassler, DAOM, L.Ac., and Executive Director Christine Cronin, DAOM, L.Ac., described the effects of their work around the world, from New Orleans after Hurricane Katrina, to Haiti after an earthquake, to communities consumed by California fires, to war-torn Ukraine. According to Cassler and Cronin, acupuncture downshifts the body's stress response and facilitates responsiveness in the cerebral cortex, which is responsible for memory, reasoning, decision-making, intelligence, and emotion, among other things. Acupuncture "helps these patients focus, solve problems, become more resilient, and move forward to rebuild their lives. . . At Acupuncturists Without Borders, we call this the Medicine of Peace — with Peace defined as a return to calm and tranquility."

Lifting depression and calming anxiety

Many adults in the United States experience the mental health conditions of anxiety and depression, according to the APA. People can experience the two disorders independently, but they often occur simultaneously.

Depression and anxiety can also coincide with other conditions, such as pain, eating disorders, heart disease, and cancer. So, healthcare providers and researchers have the tricky task of trying to separate depression and anxiety from each other and *comorbidities* (simultaneous presence of two or more diseases or medical conditions in one patient). During my episodes, I exhibited symptoms of both depression and anxiety. At times, one was more dominant than the other.

Understanding the disorders

In 2021, an estimated 21 million adults (aged over 18 years) and 5 million adolescents (aged 12–17 years) had at least one major depressive episode. Anxiety comes in a variety of forms based on the source of the anxiety, such as an irrational fear of open spaces, crowds, or leaving your home. Researchers estimate that one-third of adolescents and adults (aged 13 years and over) will suffer an anxiety disorder at some time in their lives.

Healthcare providers diagnose a major depressive episode when someone exhibits five of the following symptoms over a two-week period:

>> Consistently low mood

>> Lack of interest in formerly pleasurable activities

>> Feelings of guilt or worthlessness

>> Lack of energy

>> Poor concentration

>> Change in appetite

>> Either slow movement or hyperactive movement

>> Sleep difficulties

>> Thoughts of suicide

Anxiety and depressive disorders go beyond worry and sadness to the point that a person can't function, in degrees from mild to severe. An example of mild impairment involves difficulty concentrating, while severe impairment means you have difficulty doing anything at all. During my episodes, my impairment ranged from not being able to read to not being able to fry an egg.

TCM treatment options

Left untreated or unacknowledged, anxiety and depression can reduce a person to a shell of themselves, result in poor or irrational decisions, or lead to dangerous behavior towards oneself or others. The costs and consequences on an individual level include financial instability because of a person's inability to perform at work; reckless spending; development of chronic diseases; and broken relation-ships with partners, family, and friends.

On the societal level, anxiety and depression represent a high economic burden. A September 2023 article in the *Journal of Affective Disorders* cites that anxiety is estimated to contribute to 30 percent of the total medical costs for all mental health disorders. Finding effective, cost-efficient treatment options will not only save public and private dollars but will ease the pain of those suffering from these disorders and the anguish of their loved ones.

Researchers have examined TCM treatments for anxiety and depression quite extensively, although because TCM treatments are individualized, researchers don't have any conclusive (meaning repeatable) findings for every treatment yet. Here's a brief list of therapies that provide the following benefits, according to a few more definitive studies:

>> **Acupuncture:** Reduces the severity of depression as well as the side effects of conventional pharmaceuticals when used as a complementary therapy and seems to lower the frequency of relapses or lengthen the time of remission.

>> **Tai chi:** Studies of tai chi show its potential for improving emotional health and mental function because of its effects on the *prefrontal cortex* (the front section of the brain, which, among its many functions, is involved in personality and emotions) based on functional magnetic resonance imaging (fMRI) studies.

>> **Qigong:** Activates the parasympathetic nervous system (which controls the rest and relax functions) and lowers cortisol levels, both of which can help treat anxiety and depression.

IN THIS CHAPTER

» **Treating male and female infertility**

» **Achieving a healthy pregnancy**

» **Combining TCM with Western fertility treatments**

» **Managing labor, delivery, and aftercare**

» **Looking for reproductive health credentials**

Chapter **9**

Supporting Reproduction

aving children may seem an expected part of the human experience. But some people who want to have kids face a challenging path to parenthood. Research shows that TCM can help people conceive, improve their fertility, or experience a safe and healthy birth and delivery, wherever they are in their reproductive journey. TCM can help balance hormones, regulate the menstrual cycle, decrease stress responses, elevate endorphins, increase blood flow to reproductive organs, and improve reproductive organ functions. But not just research gives me faith in the promise of TCM: I know from my personal experience and the stories of colleagues that TCM can relieve suffering and restore hope to many potential and current parents.

In this chapter, I explore the role that Traditional Chinese Medicine (TCM) plays in supporting the reproductive process, from pre-conception to implantation to birth. I also discuss how TCM improves reproductive health, increases the potential for conception, minimizes risks for a difficult birth, and helps with postpartum medical issues.

Improving Reproductive Health

Whether or not you intend to have children, your reproductive system (the organs, glands, hormones, and so on involved in having sex and producing a baby) and its health play a critical part in your long-term well-being. Don't worry — the following sections don't include any biology and anatomy lessons. Instead, I focus on the most common reproductive issues that affect people who are designated male at birth (DMAB) or who are designated female at birth (DFAB).

Boosting male fertility

Infertility among men or DMAB people contributes to about half of the infertility issues overall, but infertility research predominantly focuses on females. Recent research indicates that semen quality has declined over the last 40 years, with a larger decline in industrialized countries. *Semen quality* generally refers to three issues, which are illustrated in Figure 9-1:

>> **Low sperm count or concentration:** The more swimmers available to travel upstream to the egg, the higher the chance that one will make it inside the egg. A low sperm count reduces those chances.

>> **Overabundance of abnormal sperm:** In any batch of cookies, you likely end up with some odd shapes. When it comes to sperm, every batch typically has a high percentage of abnormally shaped ones, but if that number goes over 96 percent, it can lead to infertility (because shape affects the ability of the sperm to penetrate and fertilize the egg).

>> **Decreased or lack of sperm *motility* (movement):** Regardless of number, if the sperm don't or can't swim in a straight line to their target, that limits the number of potential shots on goal.

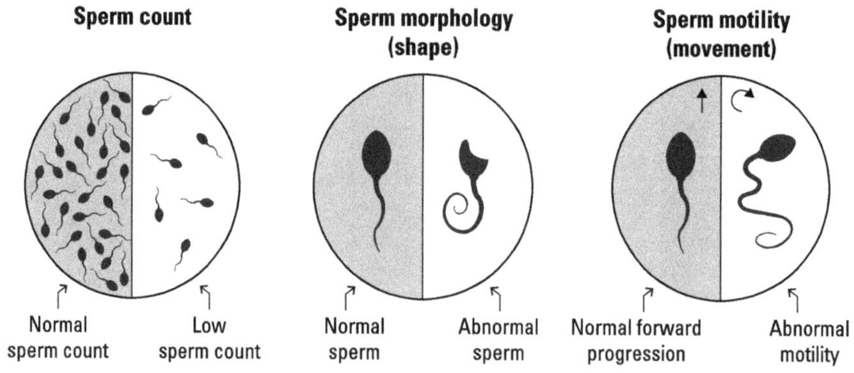

Sperm count		Sperm morphology (shape)		Sperm motility (movement)	
Normal sperm count	Low sperm count	Normal sperm	Abnormal sperm	Normal forward progression	Abnormal motility

FIGURE 9-1: Semen quality commonly involves the amount, shape, and movement of sperm.

Based on existing research, acupuncture and Traditional Chinese Herbs (TCH) can enhance the effectiveness of Western male infertility treatments. Acupuncture can increase both sperm concentration and motility through its effects on the *endocrine system* (the glands and organs that produce hormones regulating your body functions).

This is not a comprehensive discussion of all the factors that affect male fertility. Genetic or hormonal disorders, medical conditions like diabetes, infections, and cancer treatments can play a role in male infertility.

Some studies report that acupuncture regulates levels of follicle-stimulating hormone (FSH) and luteinizing hormone (LH). For men or DMAB people, FSH turns on the production of *testosterone* (in simplest terms, the hormone that tells the body to develop as a male) at puberty and kick-starts sperm production in adulthood. LH in men or DMAB people acts as the chemical messenger that says, "Get ready to reproduce." Think of FSH as the engine and LH as the key. You need to have the right levels of both at the right times for fertility.

Additional research indicates that acupuncture can also alleviate inflammation, which has a negative impact on sperm quality, and improve *testicular micro-circulation* (the movement of blood and nutrient supply to the testes). Acupuncture can also help prevent the immune system from sending anti-sperm antibodies to eliminate sperm that it identifies as invaders.

Specific TCH formulas and individual TCH also show promise in addressing the same issues.

Other TCM therapies, such as gua sha or Qigong, can reduce inflammation, improve overall balance in the body, and relieve sexual performance anxiety by promoting relaxation.

The World Journal of Men's Health has suggested that TCM's focus on overall improvement of the body and the condition and function of the testes has "effects on multiple targets, systems, and pathways to improve sperm parameters and the pregnancy rate." This focus on overall health also includes other aspects of a TCM practitioner's practice, such as nutrition and lifestyle counseling and supplement recommendations. (Please see Chapter 11 for some basic TCM nutrition tips.) While these aren't specific TCM tools, these aspects reflect the "whole-person" approach that is central to TCM.

Addressing female infertility

As noted in the preceding section, difficult conception can be equally attributed to either partner. But women or DFAB (designated female at birth) people have an infinitely more complex process than men or DMAB (designated male at birth) people because they not only supply the egg, but they carry and deliver the baby, too.

There are two kinds of female infertility:

>> **Primary infertility:** Involves someone who has never been pregnant and can't get pregnant after trying for six months (if older than 35) or one year (if younger than 35). According to the Office on Women's Health (within the U.S. Department of Health and Human Services), primary infertility affects 19 percent (or almost one out of five) of women or DFAB people between 15 and 49 years old.

>> **Secondary infertility:** When someone can't get pregnant again after at least one successful pregnancy and birth, which occurs in about 6 percent of women or DFAB people.

Although not classified, medical professionals may consider someone who can get pregnant but can't stay pregnant (someone who experiences early pregnancy loss) as infertile.

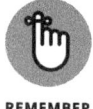

REMEMBER

Many things can contribute to infertility in women or DFAB people, such as age, hormonal imbalances, other health/medical conditions, lifestyle (such as smoking or alcohol consumption), and/or environmental factors (exposure to toxins or infections).

Specific infertility issues

The most common issues that contribute to female infertility involve the following, which are illustrated in Figure 9-2:

>> **Ovulation:** Not producing and releasing eggs regularly (somehow, the supply train isn't running on schedule); known as the *ovarian factor*.

>> **Uterus:** When the organ in which the egg makes its home is damaged in some way, making it inadequately equipped or structured to protect and sustain the egg for the term of the pregnancy; known as the *uterine factor*. Fibroids, endometriosis, scar tissue, or polyps can cause this.

>> **Egg count and quality:** Every woman or DFAB person is born with a finite number of eggs, and they may run out too soon; called *low ovarian reserve* (or low egg count).

Also, some eggs in the batch may be abnormal and, therefore, cannot be fertilized.

>> **Fallopian tubes:** A faulty connection between where the eggs are produced and where the eggs are deposited (because of pelvic adhesions, for example). Sperm also take their shots at fertilization in the fallopian tubes. This is known as the *tubal factor.*

>> **Irregular hormone levels:** Since hormones are responsible for putting the whole process in motion, it stands to reason that any hormonal disorders will have an impact on fertility. The next section provides a brief overview of the role of some of these hormones.

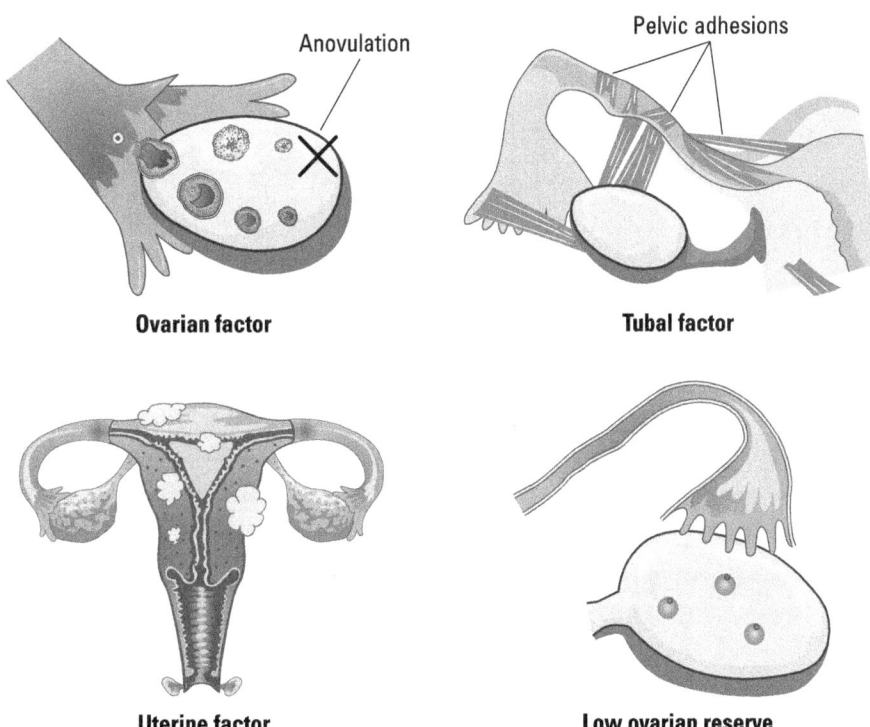

FIGURE 9-2: In addition to hormone levels, these factors can play a role in female fertility.

Anovulation

Pelvic adhesions

Ovarian factor

Tubal factor

Uterine factor

Low ovarian reserve

Research suggests that acupuncture and TCH can help with the following:

>> Relieve stress and frustration from trying to conceive

>> Increase blood (and nutrient) flow to the uterine lining for sustainable egg implantation

>> Increase blood (and nutrient) flow to other reproductive organs

>> Regulate the menstrual cycle

>> Improve thyroid gland function (if this gland is producing too little or too much of the hormones needed for reproduction)

Activating hormones

In women or DFAB people, FSH and LH trigger the ovaries at puberty to begin producing estrogen, which causes physical changes, such as breast development and menstruation. During menstruation, FSH signals the ovaries to develop the eggs, and LH signals the ovaries to release them.

Estrogen and testosterone play flipped roles in female and male reproductive processes, as shown in Table 9-1. The balance and counterbalance of these hormones fit right into TCM Yin-Yang theory (see Chapter 2).

TABLE 9-1   ## Estrogen and Testosterone at Work

Gender	Estrogen	Testosterone
Female/DFAB	Stimulates the development of female reproductive organs	Enhances the sex drive
Male/DMAB	Impacts the sex drive and the ability to have an erection	Stimulates the development of male reproductive organs

In a fascinating interview published in *The Journal of Acupuncture & Integrative Medicine*, now-retired TCM fertility expert Dr. Ann Wang, CMD, L.Ac., discussed one well-studied and used TCH formula called *Zi Shen Yu Tai Wan*. It improves *ovarian reserve* (the number of eggs left in your ovaries) by increasing FSH and LH levels. One study compared this TCH formula to hormone replacement therapy (HRT) and demonstrated that TCH treatment had equal effectiveness to HRT, with few or no adverse reactions (unlike HRT, whose subjects reported breast swelling and pain, as well as nausea and vomiting).

Zi Shen Yu Tai Wan is based on a Qing Dynasty formula (*Shou Tai Wan*) that was modified in the late 1960s by Dr. Luo Yuankai, a renowned Chinese fertility doctor and cofounder of Guangdong University of Chinese Medicine. The Chinese Ministry of Public Health recognized Luo for developing this modification and another formula for ovulation. Wang started practicing in the U.S. in 1994 and opened the Integrative Medicine Center in Ithaca, New York, in 2002. Through her work, Wang found that Western patients had more emotional and mental stress that contributed to poor egg quality and blood circulation to the ovaries, which affected ovarian reserve. To address this, Wang developed a newer variation designed for Western patients called *Fertile Tonic* for the TCM herbal company, Treasure of the East.

Treating fertility-related conditions

Acupuncture and TCH can help address conditions that relate to fertility, such as:

>> **Fibroids:** Noncancerous growths in uterine muscle tissue (see Figure 9-2)

>> **Endometriosis:** Cells from the uterine lining growing outside the uterus (refer to Figure 9-2)

>> **Polycystic ovary syndrome (PCOS):** Hormonal imbalance that affects egg production and release

>> **Side effects from fertility medications/treatments:** Including nausea, vomiting, headaches, and hot flashes or night sweats

>> **Recurrent miscarriage:** Repeated early pregnancy loss

>> **Menstrual disorders:** Including absence of periods, painful periods, heavy bleeding, irregular periods, and premenstrual syndrome

Regardless of the cause, research — and both Western and TCM practitioners — find that two heads are better than one in helping women and DFAB individuals conceive and carry safely and successfully. A number of studies published since 2019 have found that acupuncture and TCH combined with Western fertility treatments increased pregnancy and live birth rates compared to Western treatments alone.

Promoting a Healthy Pregnancy

According to a 2023 article published in the journal *Reproductive Sciences*, 1 million out of 5 million (20 percent of) pregnancies in the U.S. end in *miscarriage* (a loss before 20 weeks of gestation), and over 20,000 pregnancies end in *stillbirth* (a loss at or after 20 weeks). These losses have devastating physical and emotional consequences.

In addition to addressing infertility, practitioners have used TCM to support full-term gestation and prevent premature birth for centuries. As one of my professors explained in his analogy about reproduction: To produce a healthy crop, you need high-quality seeds; deep, rich soil; consistent care and nourishment; and proper, timely harvesting.

I discuss the seeds and soil aspects in the section "Improving Reproductive Health," earlier in this chapter, which focuses on male and female infertility. TCM treats care and feeding no differently, regardless of whether someone is pregnant or not. The goal is always to support and maintain health. During pregnancy, the goal is to prevent or minimize fetal and maternal distress in every way possible — acupuncture, *moxibustion* (burning dried mugwort near points on the body), herbs and nutrition, movement, and massage.

To put it mildly, no one thinks of pregnancy as an easy or comfortable state. The Cleveland Clinic lists over 15 pregnancy discomforts, including fatigue and lack of bladder control; a TCM practitioner treats each of these discomforts as a condition of its own. But when I consider what a pregnant person probably considers the most distressing symptoms of pregnancy, here's what comes to mind:

>> Pain

>> Nausea and vomiting

>> Anxiety or depression

Together or separate, each symptom has the potential to start a chain of problems that interfere with care and feeding, and even threaten the lives of both parent and child. For example, all three of the issues in the preceding list can decrease appetite, which may keep someone from getting the nutrients that they need to stay healthy. Similarly, all three issues can increase blood pressure, which in turn can create bigger risks, such as *preeclampsia* (a serious blood pressure condition that can develop during pregnancy).

TCM's effectiveness in relieving pain is well documented (see Chapter 7). Several studies in the *British Medical Journal* show that acupuncture can significantly relieve pain, specifically during pregnancy. The same group of studies found that acupuncture improved the quality of life for pregnant people and had no negative effects on newborns.

Scientific evidence also indicates that acupuncture and other TCM therapies calm the nervous system, release *endorphins* (the feel-good hormones), and balance hormones to ease nausea, vomiting, and anxiety. And because TCM therapies don't involve pharmaceuticals, few to no side effects can potentially harm a pregnancy.

WARNING

As in Western medicine, TCM doesn't recommend (or outright forbid) a practitioner from using certain approaches (such as specific acupuncture points, TCH, and TCM techniques) if a patient is pregnant. Licensed TCM practitioners know what to avoid.

Major hospital systems recognize the advantages of TCM and offer it in conjunction with Western obstetric and gynecological care, including the University of California, San Francisco; Stanford Health Care; the University of Pittsburgh Medical Center; Oregon Health & Science University; the University of California, Los Angeles; New York University Langone Health; Henry Ford Health (Michigan); and University Hospitals Connor Whole Health (Ohio), among others.

TIP

Ideally, a patient should start TCM treatments three to four months before they plan to try to get pregnant or before they start any fertility treatments.

Using TCM to Support Assisted Reproduction Technology

Because people often wait to have children until they're older, the window of conception narrows, so many turn to assisted reproduction technology (ART) as a means to an end. A 2019 study on the use of ART in the U.S. found a steady increase in ART use and births because of ART since 1995. You can find various ART techniques out there, including *intrauterine insemination* (in which doctors place sperm directly into the uterus), but the most common type of ART is *in vitro fertilization* (IVF), in which timing and science help overcome biological obstacles.

IVF involves a complicated sequence of events that must take place in a window of time called an *IVF cycle,* which follows these basic steps:

1. **Fertility medications stimulate the ovaries.**

2. **Doctors retrieve eggs from the woman's ovaries with a needle.**

   Alternatively, the process can use donor eggs.

3. **Doctors fertilize the egg in a lab.**

   In vitro translates as "in a laboratory."

4. **Doctors transfer the embryo to the uterus through a catheter.**

   If a woman becomes pregnant, they proceed with prenatal care.

Treating with acupuncture

Acupuncture is the most studied technique among the TCM therapies used in conjunction with IVF. As of 2019, researchers wrote reports on 40 clinical trials. Depending on the person and their fertility team, they can use acupuncture during an IVF cycle or in preparation for IVF. During the IVF cycle, treatments may start at Step 1 (see the preceding section) to encourage blood flow to the ovaries and uterus and to lower stress levels. Then, at Step 4, on the embryo transfer (ET) day, the patient receives treatment immediately before and after (within 30 minutes) the transfer procedure based on a protocol developed by German gynecologist Dr. Wolfgang Paulus in the early 2000s.

However, new research presented at the 76th Scientific Congress of the American Society for Reproductive Medicine in 2020 showed that immediate post-transfer treatment was not clinically effective. While the Paulus Protocol is still used, many ABORM practitioners have adjusted their protocol to treatment within 24 hours before ET and another treatment 5–7 days after ET. While a patient is taking IVF medication, their TCM practitioner may not prescribe any TCH (see the next section).

However, a TCM practitioner might use *moxibustion* (burning dried mugwort near acupuncture points or near inserted acupuncture needles) to heighten the effect of those acupuncture points. The TCM practitioner can even teach the patient how to use *moxa* (dried mugwort) at home (without the needles, of course). Alternatively, the practitioner can teach their patient to apply *ear seeds* (tiny adhesive acacia seeds that can be affixed to specific points on the ear). (See Chapter 5 for more information on these techniques.)

Deciding when to use acupuncture

In preparation for IVF, practitioners recommend acupuncture for three to four months before the patient starts taking the IVF medication. TCH can help prepare the system for the upcoming cycle, depending on the patient's condition and consultation with their supervising physician. Some patients will stop taking the TCH after they start medication, while others may continue with TCH in conjunction with the ovarian stimulation medication. These decisions are all discussed and determined by the patient's care team as part of their treatment plan. The TCM practitioner integrates acupuncture during the IVF cycle (as discussed in the preceding section).

Overall, research shows that acupuncture can help with IVF in the following ways:

>> Reduces the side effects from IVF medications and enhances responsiveness to these medications

>> Enriches the uterine lining by improving blood flow to the uterus

>> Eases the stress and anxiety associated with the ART process

>> Lowers the risk of miscarriage and *ectopic* (outside the uterus) pregnancy, thereby improving chances of live birth

Lending a Hand During and After Birth

For people who have never had a baby or haven't helped deliver one, their understanding of the birthing process may be limited to what they've seen on TV or in the movies: huffing and puffing, pain and pushing, and then out pops a precious little package ready to be swaddled and cuddled.

AUTHOR SAYS

I was blessed to be in the room when my godson was born, and the process looked and sounded excruciating. (A coworker of mine described her birth process as pushing a piano through a transom window.) I had no idea what was happening to my dear friend's body that made it possible for my godson to emerge safely and for her to recover smoothly. Thankfully, I was also clueless about what could have gone woefully wrong.

Easing labor and delivery

I was lucky enough to receive knowledge and wisdom from Dr. Claudia Citkovitz, Ph.D., M.S., L.Ac., whom I met through my alma mater, the American College of Traditional Chinese Medicine, and learned from at conferences and in continuing education seminars. As a leading TCM authority and researcher in labor and delivery, as well as stroke recovery, Dr. Citkovitz teaches, lectures, and publishes extensively in the U.S. and Europe.

Several studies suggest that TCM improves labor and birth experiences. Depending on the patient and their specific condition, Dr. Citkovitz recommends acupressure, tui na, moxibustion, movement, and breathwork (which you can read about in Chapter 5) to provide what she describes as comfort, flow, and balance during labor. Whether they reduce pain, stimulate or smooth contractions, soften the cervix, or provide a boost of energy, these TCM techniques can ease the birthing process for both parent and child. Better yet, anyone on the birthing team can learn these techniques — doctor or midwife, partner or family member.

Turning a breech baby

It might sound like an old wives' tale, but a 2023 Cochrane review (a systematic review of research published in the Cochrane Database) of 13 studies that included 2,181 patients found that moxibustion treatment before the 37th week of pregnancy probably reduces the chance of breech presentation. (You can read about moxibustion in Chapter 5.) It's *not* guaranteed, but I referred one patient who was breech to a TCM reproductive specialist (see the section "Certifying a Specialty," later in this chapter). The baby turned after one treatment, and the patient safely delivered two weeks later.

Breech presentation means that the baby is positioned with their bottom pointing toward the cervix. Most babies turn head-down before labor starts, but some don't turn naturally. A baby in breech presentation has a more difficult time emerging from the womb without serious complications, such as dislocated or broken bones, a trapped or stuck head, or issues with the umbilical cord.

Breastfeeding

After birth, breastfeeding can offer positive short- and long-term health benefits for the baby, including better nutrition and enhanced immunity. Common breast-feeding difficulties include low milk production and breast swelling and soreness.

A 2024 review and meta-analysis (a research method that combines or summarizes data from multiple independent studies on the same subject or topic) found that TCM can improve lactation and breast fullness, making breastfeeding more comfortable and more likely to occur. Researchers analyzed 20 studies that included gua sha, cupping, moxibustion, and ear seeds (see Chapter 5), as well as acupressure (see Chapter 12). Combined with acupuncture at points tailored to individual patient constitutions, these noninvasive techniques appeared to help increase milk production and decrease *mastitis* (breast inflammation). The study also found that the TCM therapy was more effective if the practitioner initiated it within 24 hours of delivery and continued it for at least one week.

Managing postpartum depression

Sometimes dismissed as "the baby blues," postpartum depression (PPD) is the most common complication after birth. According to World Health Organization (WHO) data, the likelihood of experiencing mental disorders after delivery is

13 percent. In developed countries such as the U.S., the likelihood rises to almost 20 percent. That's one in five new child bearers feeling like something is wrong at one of the most memorable and special times in their lives. Both parent and child face wide-ranging risks if PPD occurs.

The standard Western medical treatment for PPD includes medication and psychotherapy. Although both types of treatments can certainly help, not everyone has access to these treatments. Others have concerns about the side effects of antidepressants, and some simply don't respond well to medication.

Practitioners have used TCM — including acupuncture, Traditional Chinese Herbs (TCH), massage, and movement (check out Chapters 4 and 5 for discussion of these treatments) — to treat depressive disorders for thousands of years. Increasing scientific evidence supports TCM's efficacy in this area. (See Chapter 8 for more information about using TCM to treat depression.)

For PPD specifically, TCM offers a viable complementary or alternative approach. A 2022 review published in *Frontiers in Neuroendocrinology* suggests that combining TCH with *paroxetine* (an antidepressant more commonly known by the brand name Paxil) can have a clinical effect, with patients reporting improvement in symptoms. (*Clinical effect* is different from *clinical significance*, which indicates measurable changes.) A 2023 review and meta-analysis of 35 trials that involved 2,848 participants showed that combining a modified version of a classic TCM formula with Western medical treatment led to lower Hamilton Rating Scale for Depression (HAM-D) scores and higher effectiveness than Western medicine alone.

Certifying a Specialty

Historically, people have used TCM extensively for reproductive health. But only recently have medical professionals recognized TCM's role in reproductive health by offering specialized training and certification in this area. Leading practitioners in Chinese reproductive medicine founded the international nonprofit organization Acupuncture and TCM Board of Reproductive Medicine (ABORM) in 2007 to establish a certification program and examination that demonstrates a practitioner's advanced knowledge in both TCM and Western reproductive health.

To become a certified Fellow of ABORM, you don't have to be a TCM practitioner. Medical doctors, naturopaths, nurses, physical therapists, and others in the field of reproductive health can receive certification. The skills of an ABORM practitioner extend beyond TCM and integrate the unique perspectives of many different branches of medicine.

TIP

Trained to collaborate with other clinicians, ABORM practitioners can offer patients the best of both worlds, giving them the best chance to safely conceive and deliver a baby. To find an ABORM practitioner, you can visit the ABORM website's Find a Practitioner page at www.aborm.org/find-a-practitioner.

Chapter **10**

Supporting Cancer Treatment

et me start with the good news: According to the American Cancer Society, the risk of dying from cancer has steadily declined in recent years, in part because of a decrease in the number of smokers, early cancer screenings, and advancements in cancer treatments.

But here's the bad news: The number of cancer cases is rising for six of the ten most common cancers: breast, prostate, endometrial, pancreatic, kidney, and skin (melanoma, specifically). (Lung, colon and rectum, and bladder cancers, and non-Hodgkin's lymphoma, a cancer of the blood, round out the top 10.) In 2024, over 2 million new cancer cases were reported in the U.S. for the first time. That's almost 5,500 cancer diagnoses a day. Sadly, over 618,000 cancer deaths were projected for the same year, which works out to more than 1,600 cancer deaths each day.

I don't know about you, but I've lost family and friends to cancer and have others fighting it right now. The fight involves one or more treatment options, including surgery, chemotherapy, radiotherapy, targeted therapy, and immunotherapy. If you've experienced these treatments or watched a loved one experience them, you know it's no walk in the park. In fact, it's a brutal test of endurance through a gauntlet of side effects.

In this chapter, I focus on how Traditional Chinese Medicine (TCM) therapies can support patients in fighting cancer and successfully emerge from treatment less battered and worn out than when they started. As part of this discussion, I share a case study: a patient I treated when I was an intern, where I used TCM diagnosis and treatment to counteract the side effects from her cancer treatments.

Recognizing TCM Cancer-Treatment Therapies

TCM has been used for centuries to treat different cancers in China and other East Asian countries. The earliest reference to a tumor (*liu*) was found on oracle bone engravings and tortoise shells from the Shang Dynasty (16th–11th century BCE). Classical texts, such as the *Huang Di Nei Jing* (see Chapter 4) of the Warring Period (475–221 BCE), describe how these tumors are formed. My summary of the *Nei Jing* description, in the simplest TCM terms (see Chapter 2), is as follows:

Tumors form when Qi and Blood don't move or become stuck (this is called Qi and Blood Stagnation). This lack of circulation leads to Excess (too much) Cold because good circulation keeps Qi and Blood warm and flowing. The buildup of Cold creates an opposing Heat response that manifests as fever. Instead of releasing the Cold and the Stagnation, the Heat ends up "cooking" the Cold mass of Qi and Blood, which damages the flesh and bones and eventually reaches the organs. Without proper Qi and Blood circulation, the organ systems can't function normally, which ultimately leads to death.

TECHNICAL
STUFF

TCM uses individualized treatment, even for cancer. With more research and development being focused on immunotherapy that targets specific cell markers, it seems to me that Western medicine is coming around to a similar approach.

Any combination of the tools in the TCM therapy kit, which I describe in Chapters 4 and 5 — acupuncture, Traditional Chinese Herbs (TCH), *moxibustion* (burning dried mugwort near points on the body), cupping, tui na, Qigong, tai chi, and dietary and lifestyle advice — can provide tailored, whole-person care in a cancer battle. To show how a practitioner can use TCM cancer-treatment therapy to complement Western medicine cancer treatment, I share a case study, where I applied TCM diagnosis and acupuncture to counteract a patient's side effects from cancer treatment.

Presenting a Case Study: Ovarian Cancer

The patient was a 52-year-old who self-identified as female. For the sake of our story, I'll call her Mary. Mary was diagnosed with Stage 4 ovarian cancer and began a series of nine chemotherapy sessions within two months of diagnosis. (Figure 10-1 illustrates the four stages of ovarian cancer.)

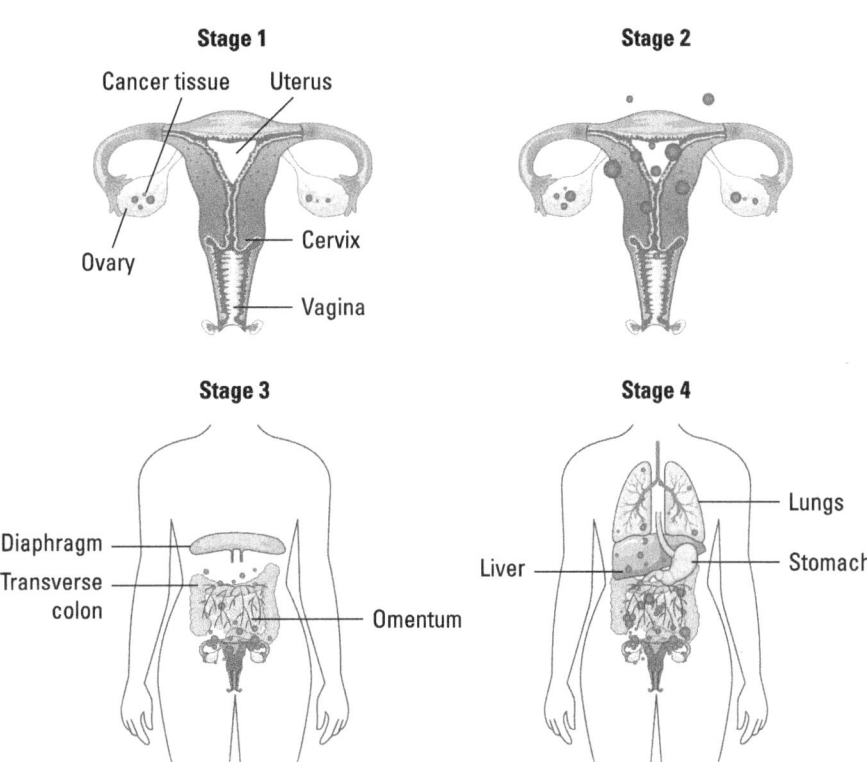

FIGURE 10-1: The progression of ovarian cancer is tracked over four stages.

According to the American Cancer Society, ovarian cancer is one of the leading causes of cancer death among women in the U.S., and an estimated 12,730 women will die from it in 2025. Because this cancer typically shows up late, it's often diagnosed after progressing significantly. The five-year survival rate for ovarian cancer depends on the type of cell that developed abnormally and the stage at which medical professionals detect and start to treat it, but it ranges 50–92 percent.

Navigating the Western medicine approach

In very basic terms, cancer develops when cells grow and multiply out of control — not the norm. The norm is a nonstop production line, with cells copying themselves to restock the supply needed to replace old or damaged ones. In the cell factory that is your body, each cell gets assigned to a specific department, such as the bone builders, the skin surfacers, or the muscle makers. In addition to having jobs, most cells have a built-in shelf life. When a cell dies (known as *apoptosis*), another one glides in without a hitch in the system. This amazing process produces an estimated 300 billion cells each day (oh, if we had a dollar for every cell . . .), and this process keeps going until our own time comes.

But for various hard-to-explain reasons, not every cell comes out of the factory up to par. They might go to the wrong department; they might not be properly formed to do the job that they're assigned to; or they might not die when they should. These misfit cells gather and form tumors (or masses or lumps) that interfere with normal body functions, and chaos follows. To illustrate, here's a comparison of normal cell growth (see Figure 10-2) and abnormal cell growth (see Figure 10-3).

NORMAL CELL DEVELOPMENT

FIGURE 10-2: Every normal cell multiplies into a divided cell to form healthy tissue.

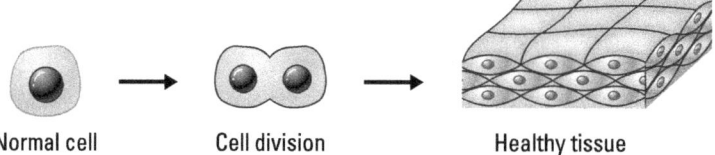

Normal cell   Cell division   Healthy tissue

ABNORMAL CELL GROWTH

FIGURE 10-3: In cancer, a normal cell experiences an abnormal change. It proceeds to multiply as cancerous cells, which form a cancerous tumor.

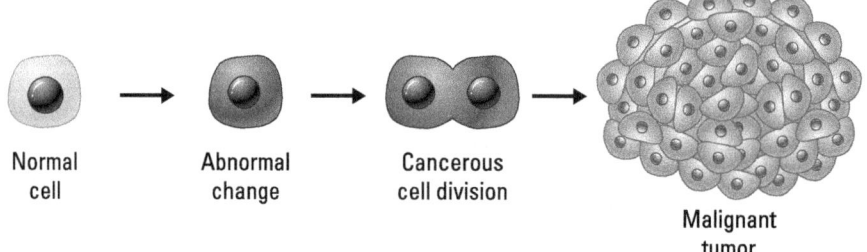

Normal cell   Abnormal change   Cancerous cell division   Malignant tumor

Western diagnostics discover these cancerous cells through physical examination, such as feeling for lumps, and using blood tests and imaging, such as computed tomography (CT) scans, positron emission tomography (PET) scans, and magnetic resonance imaging (MRI).

Depending on the type and stage of ovarian cancer, the most common forms of treatment are surgery and chemotherapy. However, Western medicine also uses radiation, hormones, targeted drugs, and immune therapies to treat ovarian and other cancers.

In Mary's case, blood tests and imaging determined her diagnosis. In her initial phase of treatment, Mary received a pair of drugs every week (instead of every three weeks) in an approach called *dose-dense chemotherapy.* The strategy involved administering the same amount of medication in one week that, in standard therapy, she would receive every three weeks to maintain a constant level of the medication in her system.

Mary's two drugs were paclitaxel and carboplatin. As a one-two punch, paclitaxel attacks the cells when they're in the middle of dividing so that they can't multiply, and carboplatin scrambles genetic material in the cells to keep those cells from reproducing.

Defining the TCM diagnosis

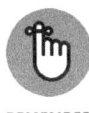

REMEMBER

For a TCM diagnostic approach, I apply the concepts discussed in Chapter 2, including the Vital Three (Qi, Blood, and Body Fluid), the Eight Balances (Yin and Yang, Hot and Cold, Deficiency and Excess, and Exterior and Interior), and the Five Elements (Earth, Wind, Water, Wood, and Fire). Please refer to that chapter if you need more information about these theories.

In the simplest TCM terms, cancerous tumors form when one or more of the Vital Three substances don't circulate properly. Poor circulation can lead to a buildup that becomes a mass that throws the body out of balance. Any number of environmental (external) or emotional (internal) pathogenic factors can cause poor circulation.

To diagnose Mary's case (or any case, for that matter), a TCM practitioner needs to find out which of the Eight Balances are out of whack, what pathogenic factors play a part in the imbalance, and how these factors are creating a Qi problem.

Table 11-1 shows the Five Elements categories that I referenced to assess Mary's case, which are examined in the sections that follow.

TABLE 11-1   **The Five Elements and Their Characteristics**

Items	Earth	Metal	Water	Wood	Fire
Organs	Spleen and Stomach	Lung and Large Intestine	Kidney and Urinary Bladder	Liver and Gallbladder	Heart and Small Intestine
Emotion	Worry	Grief or sadness	Fear	Anger	Joy
Actions and Functions	Reproducing; changing or transforming; receiving	Dispersing and descending; harvesting or holding	Storing, moistening, flowing downwards	Growing, ascending, and flourishing	Expanding, evaporating, and flaring
Environmental Pathogen	Dampness (Yin)	Dryness (Yang)	Cold (Yin)	Wind (Yang)	Heat (Yang)

Environmental pathogens

I deliberately skipped discussing environmental pathogens in detail in Chapter 2 because there's only so much a person can retain at one time. It took two parts of Fundamental Theory and three parts of TCM Diagnosis for me to grasp these concepts, let alone explain them. But they are relevant to this case study, so I'm attempting to describe them here.

The environmental pathogens listed in the mini-table above and the larger table in Chapter 2 refer to pathogenic factors that contribute to disease. They are typically *external* pathogenic factors — attacking or invading from the outside. However, once they get inside and stay a while, they become *internal* pathogenic factors. For example, I went to a baseball game in San Francisco while the sun was out, but I didn't have a coat to wear after dark. External Cold invaded my lungs, and I developed a cough and chills the next day. Left without treatment, the external Cold can build up in my lungs to become internal Cold and manifest as pneumonia.

More than one pathogen attacking at the same time (for example, Dampness and Cold manifesting as diarrhea and stiff joints) or one pathogen creating other pathogens (Cold becoming Wind-Heat manifesting as a sore throat and high fever) are other complications a TCM practitioner will likely have to confront. It is not unusual for this to happen. No condition is static. The body and its systems are constantly changing to maintain balance or homeostasis.

TCM diagnosis is focused on the most dominant signs and symptoms that trouble you most at the time of your examination. In the example of Dampness and Cold, there are additional signs and symptoms like tongue and pulse (see Chapter 6) that will help guide the diagnosis toward the pathogen that needs to be addressed first to provide you with relief and move you toward recovery.

The following sections discuss the main characteristics and properties of the environmental pathogens, as well as present examples of symptoms that manifest when the pathogens are at work in the body.

DAMPNESS (*SHI*)

In various textbooks, Dampness is described as wet, heavy, slow, and turbid (cloudy). It builds up or accumulates. It sticks around and is pliable but hard to break up. Dampness can combine with Cold or Heat. I associate Damp-Cold with an Irish bog and Damp-Heat with a Florida swamp. Neither are conditions I want to experience.

» **Yin pathogen:** A Yin pathogen is Yin in its basic nature. Looking back to Chapter 2 and the Eight Principles of balance, the foremost pair of principles is Yin and Yang. So, the characteristics of Dampness that classify it as Yin are slow, heavy, cloudy, and moist.

» **Point of entry:** Attacks the lower (Yin) part of the body (for example, edema in the legs).

» **Direction:** Moves downward (Yin) (for example, edema in the legs). The *Nei Jing* (see Chapter 4) states that "the lower body is the first area affected by Dampness."

» **Effects:** Obstructs or impedes Spleen Qi activities and functions, which involve turning food and water into Qi and Blood. To do this, the Spleen prefers dryness to send Qi and Blood upward (Yang) for distribution throughout the body by the lungs and heart. When the Spleen isn't right, the whole system goes wrong. Without the Spleen making enough good-quality Qi and Blood, the body becomes malnourished and weak.

» **Symptoms:** Examples include dull, heavy feeling in the head; heavy and sore limbs or joints; fullness in the chest or abdomen; loss of appetite; indigestion; nausea; abdominal edema (swelling caused by too much fluid in the abdominal tissue); muddy diarrhea; cloudy, dribbling, or incomplete urine; thick vaginal discharge; and obsessive thoughts or worrying.

DRYNESS (*ZAO*)

Dryness is a direct contrast to Dampness and represents Heat to the point of dehydration. Dryness is not a common TCM diagnosis because it is so closely related to Heat and exhibits similar symptoms.

» **Yang pathogen:** As a contrast to Dampness, Dryness is a Yang pathogen. Its Yin characteristics are dry and light.

>> **Point of entry:** Usually invades through the mouth and/or nose.

>> **Effects:** Damages Body Fluid and injures the Lung, which circulates Qi, Blood, and Body Fluid. If this circulation is disrupted, it can weaken Qi or deplete Body Fluid anywhere in the body. A typical example is asthma or being prone to catching colds.

>> **Symptoms:** Examples include dry nostrils leading to a bloody nose; dry lips, tongue, skin, and stools; dry cough; chest pain; and sudden fever.

COLD (*HAN*)

Cold in nature and the body are exactly what you think. Cold is not warm and not moving. Cold contracts and makes you want to curl up under a wool blanket. Cold to the extreme can freeze and become hard and fixed.

>> **Yin pathogen:** Cold is a Yin pathogen as the opposing nature of Heat. It slows or restricts movement like Dampness, but Cold is rigid, while Dampness is like a marshmallow. Its Yin characteristics are obvious, but they include cold, hard, immobile, and so on.

>> **Point of entry:** Often can accompany Wind (see below) into the body. Cold can also develop from poor circulation of Qi and Blood or a deficient supply of Yang, which is caused by any number of other pathologies.

>> **Path:** As a Yin pathogen, Cold can be associated with downward movement, but it may not move at all.

>> **Effects:** Impairs, restricts, or limits Yang functions in the body like warming, stimulating, and activating, which is most associated with the Kidneys; obstructs Qi, Blood, and/or Body Fluid. As one of the Eight Principles paired with Heat, Cold can temper the effects of Heat in a good way. As a contributor to illness, Cold acts against Heat or sometimes overcomes it. The *Nei Jing* states "Cold enters the [organ] channels and there is retardation of movement . . . the Qi cannot penetrate, and finally, there is pain."

>> **Symptoms:** Examples include feeling cold or actually being cold to the touch; sluggishness; pale complexion; severe, sharp, or cramping pain in limbs and joints; stiffness in limbs and joints; frequent urination; lack of libido (sexual desire); emotional detachment; and fearfulness.

WIND (*FENG*)

The Wind pathogen is much like the air that blows around us. It is wayward, quick, light, and moves almost too much. As a pathogen, it is sudden and disruptive; it comes and goes rapidly and shakes the body like it shakes leaves and branches on trees.

» **Yang pathogen:** Wind is Yang in nature, being quick, light, and active.

» **Point of entry:** Attacks and invades the upper (Yang) part of the body.

» **Path:** Moves upward and outward (Yang); migrates (wanders, comes and goes, has no fixed time or location); and changes (sudden onset and/or rapid progression/transformation).

» **Effects:** Wind is the most common cause of illness in TCM because it rarely manifests by itself and facilitates the invasion of other pathogens. The *Nei Jing* (see Chapter 4) states that "the hundred diseases develop from Wind." TCM addresses two types of Wind:

- **External Wind:** External Wind often attacks the Lung first in partnership with Heat or Cold. *Wind-Heat* shows up with a moderate or high fever, a sore throat, and maybe sweating, and *Wind-Cold* brings chills, low or no fever, and maybe fatigue.

- **Internal Wind:** If Wind penetrates deeper to become internal Wind, it attacks the Liver, which is closely associated with Blood. In TCM, when the Liver is working properly, it's the ultimate diplomat, asserting itself when needed to control the supply and movement of Blood, yet being strategic and flexible in how it collaborates with the other organs (Kidney, Spleen, and others) to keep all systems functioning. Internal Wind throws the Liver off its game.

» **Symptoms:** See the previous bullet for examples of the symptoms that can be caused by external Wind. Internal Wind examples include:

- Dizziness

- Pain that shifts in location

- Tinnitus (ringing or other noise in the ears)

- Numb limbs

- Tremors, convulsions, or twitching

- Short temper or explosive anger

- Being overly or inappropriately aggressive or forceful

HEAT (*RE*) OR FIRE (*HUO*)

In reference to pathogenic factors, Heat and Fire are almost identical. The difference is that Heat is often external and Fire is typically internal. Heat and Fire are both hot and active. Heat and Fire expand and spread and keep you out of saunas.

» **Yang pathogen:** As the partner of Cold among the Eight Principles, Heat and Fire are Yang pathogens that are critical to achieving a healthy balance in the body. If not controlled or balanced, Heat and Fire behave like they do in nature — flaring, expanding, stimulating, or moving with reckless abandon.

» **Point of entry:** As an external pathogen, Heat usually accompanies Wind or Dampness and enters through the Lungs or Spleen. As an internal pathogen, Fire can be generated by a buildup of other pathogens, like Dampness or by excessive emotions like anger.

» **Path:** Moves upward; rises and spreads (Yang).

» **Effects:** Consumes Yin and Body Fluid; accelerates Blood circulation or causes uncontrolled bleeding. Internal Fire affects the Heart and its outer protective layer, the Pericardium. Fire disrupts the Heart's function of regulating Blood flow and maintaining the Spirit (*shen*). Again, I turn to Ted Kaptchuk's *The Web That Has No Weaver* (2000, McGraw-Hill) for a better expression of the Heart's job in relation to the Spirit than I can devise: "The Heart is responsible for appropriate behavior, timely interactions, and being suitable to the context. Being respectful, helpful, thoughtful, or emotional is only virtuous when the Heart Spirit ensures that the moment is right."

» **Symptoms:** Examples of External Heat include thirst; high fever; sweating; headache; sore and dry throat; rash; feeling hot or being hot to the touch; red face and eyes; and *scanty* (less than normal amount of) or dark urine. Examples of Internal Fire include coughing up or vomiting blood; blood in urine or stool; excess menstruation; heart palpitations; insomnia; delirium; and anxiety.

Emotional factors

Although emotions are natural and healthy, TCM theory indicates that having too much emotion can upset the balance and relationships of the Five Elements because each of the Elements is associated with an emotion. A healthy expression of emotion occurs when the Elements are relating harmoniously. However, in TCM theory, emotion can stir up imbalance in the organs and channels, and vice versa. Anger can raise blood pressure, or an imbalance in the Liver can make someone more prone to anger.

When someone is facing the challenge of cancer, naturally, plenty of emotions are in play that affect the diagnosis, treatment, and outcomes in both Western medicine and TCM.

Although emotional factors are extremely relevant, I can't provide the details in this case study because Mary didn't share much of her emotional experiences with me before her cancer diagnosis or after. To read more about how TCM can be applied to help manage mental health, see Chapter 8.

AUTHOR SAYS

In hindsight, if I were a more experienced interviewer during intake, I would have been more direct in asking Mary about how she felt about her diagnosis and the cancer treatment. In my practice today, I explain at the very first session that I ask questions that might seem irrelevant to the patient's chief complaint, but that all the questions give me a more comprehensive picture of them and their health issue. I also state that they don't have to answer any questions that make them uncomfortable. If a patient returns for more treatments and I gain their trust, I will return to any questions we skipped if I think the answers will help with my diagnosis and treatment.

Assessing the Case

For my patient Mary (see the section "Presenting a Case Study: Ovarian Cancer," earlier in this chapter), I based her TCM diagnosis on an assessment of her reported symptoms and the signs that I observed from her initial intake interview and examination and at each of her three follow-up sessions.

REMEMBER

A TCM diagnosis can change based on how the patient presents (or appears) at each session. Although the initial intake is the most extensive interview and examination (see Chapter 6), the TCM practitioner conducts an abbreviated intake interview and examination at each session, so the TCM practitioner can adjust subsequent treatments based on the results of the previous session.

Reported symptoms

The following is a summary of Mary's symptoms:

>> Fatigue

- Difficulty getting out of bed

- Little energy or motivation to do things

- ❯❯ Lower abdominal pain and fullness
  - • Uterus hurts and feels like it's being pulled from below
  - • Sensation of intense contraction and release
  - • Pain comes and goes; some days no pain at all
  - • Patient feels relief from pain after urination
- ❯❯ Heat sensations
  - • Spontaneous sweating
  - • Hot flushes that felt like being on fire inside
- ❯❯ Lower back, sciatic, and neck pain
- ❯❯ Low to no appetite
- ❯❯ Sleep interrupted by pain and/or heat sensations
- ❯❯ Feelings of sadness

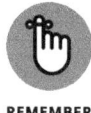

REMEMBER

Prescription and over-the-counter drugs can mask the true presentation of symptoms, so a TCM practitioner must consider the presence of medication in the system when evaluating a patient.

Observed signs

Here are some of the signs that I observed in Mary:

- ❯❯ **Behavior:** Fully mobile, despite reported fatigue; genial and pleasant demeanor; overall positive and hopeful attitude, despite her condition.
- ❯❯ **Tongue:** Generally dusky in color, but sometimes red at the tip; thin in shape; dry, with little or scanty coating (film on the surface of the tongue).
- ❯❯ **Pulse:** Bowstring (like a violin string) in first position; slippery and forceful in second position; and deep, small, and weak in third position.

REMEMBER

When taking your pulse, a TCM practitioner places their index, middle, and ring fingers along your radial artery, which runs up the thumb side of your arm. The index is the first position, the middle is the second, and the ring is the third. Each position corresponds to a specific organ or organ channel.

Chapter 6 provides more information about inspecting the tongue and pulse for diagnostic purposes. The tongue often indicates if a condition is external and acute or internal and chronic. Both tongue and pulse will provide clues about which pathogenic factor is involved, as well as which organ system or organ channel is affected.

Figuring Out the TCM Diagnosis

Based on her signs and symptoms noted in the section "Assessing the Case," earlier in this chapter, I outlined my evaluation of Mary's Eight Balances, as shown in the following list.

REMEMBER

The bold text in this list represents the dominant or more prevalent of the paired principles.

Yin or Yang

>> Lower body involvement in the ovaries [**YIN** or YANG]

>> Structural impairment to the ovaries [**YIN** or YANG]

>> Functional impairment to the ovaries [YIN or **YANG**]

Cold or Hot

>> Heat sensations COLD or **HOT**]

>> Spontaneous sweating [COLD or **HOT**]

>> Hot flushes; fire inside [COLD or **HOT**]

>> Sleep interrupted by pain and/or heat sensations [COLD or **HOT**]

>> Dusky (purplish) tongue color with red tip [COLD or **HOT**]

>> Thin, dry tongue that had little or no coating [COLD or **HOT**]

Deficiency or Excess

>> Fatigue; lack of energy [**DEFICIENCY** or EXCESS]

>> Lower abdominal pain and fullness [DEFICIENCY or **EXCESS**]

>> Heat sensations [DEFICIENCY or **EXCESS**]

>> Low back, sciatic, and neck pain [DEFICIENCY or **EXCESS**]

>> Low to no appetite [**DEFICIENCY** or EXCESS]

>> Sleep interrupted by pain and/or heat sensations [DEFICIENCY or **EXCESS**]

>> Dusky (purplish) tongue color with red tip [DEFICIENCY or **EXCESS**]

>> Thin, dry tongue that had little or no coating [**DEFICIENCY** or EXCESS]

>> Bowstring, slippery, forceful pulse [DEFICIENCY or **EXCESS**]

>> Deep, small, weak pulse [**DEFICIENCY** or EXCESS]

Interior or Exterior

>> Spontaneous sweating [INTERIOR or **EXTERIOR**]

>> Hot flushes; fire inside [**INTERIOR** or EXTERIOR]

Mary's symptoms and signs indicated a combination of imbalances. But she had more Hot than Cold and a bit more Excess than Deficiency. To cut to the chase, a deeper assessment of the pulse positions and symptoms (timing, location in the body) led to a diagnosis that amounted to a combination of two of the four Qi problems discussed in Chapter 2 — Weak Qi and Blocked Qi.

The environmental factors contributing to Mary's diagnosis are:

>> Dampness

>> Heat

Combine these two factors, and the results are a sticky, steaming swamp that becomes toxic. According to one text on integrating conventional treatment with TCM for cancer, "Qi and Blood Deficiency (Weak Qi) with knotted toxin (Blocked Qi)" manifests during Stage 4 cancer with symptoms such as fatigue, weakness, spontaneous sweating, and lower abdominal fullness and pain. Mary reported experiencing all these symptoms.

TECHNICAL STUFF

Another characterization of cancer that I encountered while treating Mary is from the publication *Supportive Cancer Care with Chinese Medicine*, edited by William C.S. Cho (2010, Springer). It states that cancer results from an imbalance that "affects the normal flow of vital energy and informational signals through the system, resulting in unchecked, prolonged stagnation (Blocked Qi) of these elements that in turn, transform normal healthy tissues in the stagnated area to morbid tissues and eventually cancerous growth."

With this analysis, I realized that to restore some kind of balance for Mary, I needed to clear Heat and resolve Dampness to help restore movement of Qi and Blood; encourage or manage the movement of Qi and Blood to clear Heat and resolve Dampness; and strengthen or fortify the Qi and Blood of the whole system.

Easing the Side Effects of Cancer Treatment

In Mary's case, her doctors prescribed chemotherapy to both halt the growth of cancer cells and outright kill the cancer cells already in her body. Unfortunately, chemotherapy also damages healthy cells, which results in a range of side effects. Sometimes these side effects are more debilitating than the effects of the cancer itself and make it difficult for the patient to tolerate or complete the treatment, which can threaten a successful treatment outcome.

Mary received her first acupuncture treatment about five days before her first scheduled chemotherapy session. The goal for her first treatment was to help her withstand anticipated side effects.

Fighting fatigue and boosting energy

Even before Mary's chemotherapy started, her number one complaint was fatigue, which interfered with her daily activities. Fatigue, which everyone feels at some time in their life, is a sign that you need to rest, and it usually goes away after you allow yourself to recharge.

Cancer-related fatigue (CRF) is an entirely different type of exhaustion. Rest doesn't help; in fact, you feel so tired that you can't fall asleep. Your arms and legs feel like 100-pound weights. You have difficulty even thinking, let alone dressing or eating. And forget about sex or intimacy. CRF affects 65 to 90 percent of patients at some time during their cancer journey, especially during the time that they receive chemotherapy and/or radiotherapy.

Usually, CRF resolves within a year of finishing treatment, but studies indicate that 20 to 30 percent of survivors continue to experience CRF symptoms for five or more years.

Treating fatigue by using acupuncture

Mary's first treatment included acupuncture that used points on her back to regulate and nourish Blood and fortify Qi; on her lower limbs to invigorate and nourish Blood, clear Heat, and support and foster Qi; on her upper limbs to strengthen Qi; and on her head to raise and *tonify* (strengthen and support) Qi.

Growing evidence shows that acupuncture is an effective intervention for CRF and fatigue, in general. A 2023 meta-analysis of 34 studies published in *Frontiers in Oncology* concluded that acupuncture was "an effective and safe strategy for alleviating cancer-related fatigue." In 2022, *Phytomedicine* published an overview of fifty-one systematic reviews with the conclusion that acupuncture was beneficial for CRF, as well as other cancer-related issues such as pain and insomnia.

A 2015 study at the Sloan Kettering Cancer Center in New York found that true acupuncture demonstrated a 36 percent improvement in fatigue levels compared to acupressure and sham acupuncture. Sham acupuncture simulates acupuncture in various ways, such as inserting needles in random points or using an instrument that might feel like a needle but isn't.

Using moxibustion, herbal formulas, and movement to treat CRF

For Mary's treatment, I applied moxibustion to specific points to nourish Blood and Qi. As you can read about in Chapter 5, moxibustion boosts the actions of individual points while also creating a state of deep relaxation.

Depending on the TCM diagnosis, TCM practitioners routinely use one of several Traditional Chinese Herbs (TCH) formulas for fatigue, targeting the root cause. But as I discuss in the section "Fighting fatigue and boosting energy," earlier in this chapter, CRF is like fatigue on steroids. One formula that I recommended for Mary features cordyceps fruiting body (*dong chong xia cao*), which TCM prescribes as a tonic ingredient that restores energy, promotes longevity, and improves quality of life (see Figure 10-4).

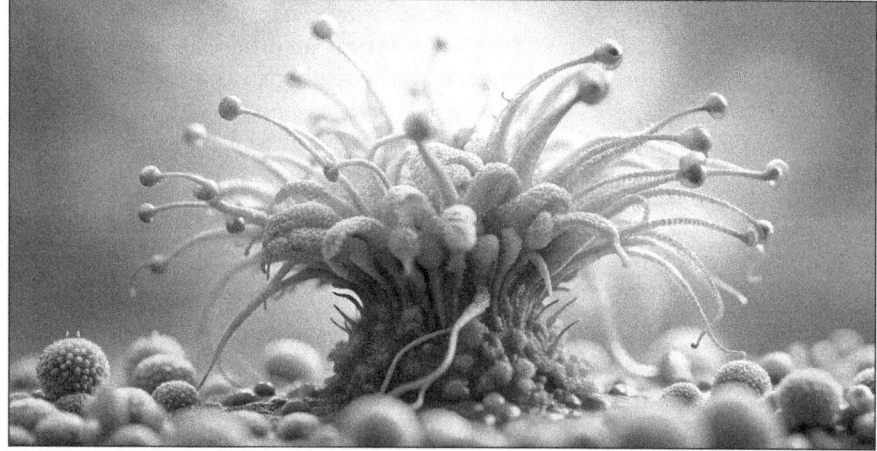

FIGURE 10-4:
Cordyceps or Chinese caterpillar fungus is described as being warm, harmonious, and tonifying.

LittleBird919/Adobe Stock Photos

Although it may seem counterintuitive for fatigue, the Guidelines for the Management of Cancer-Caused Fatigue published by the National Comprehensive Cancer Network (NCCN) recommend exercise therapy to manage fatigue symptoms in cancer patients. Tai chi and Qigong both offer gentle forms of physical movement that build strength, energy, and fitness. A number of studies from 2015 to 2020 have confirmed the efficacy of tai chi and Qigong to treat CRF. In addition to energy, strength, and fitness, these exercise therapies also improve balance, mental clarity, and relaxation.

Reducing post-treatment pain and neuropathy

Many cancer patients commonly experience pain that differs in location and character depending upon the type of cancer and the treatment plan, as well as post-treatment nerve pain (also known as *neuropathy*). The cancer's effects on her body obviously caused Mary's pain, but the chemotherapy also contributed to the pain she experienced. Mary received acupuncture both local to and *distal* to (away from) the location of pain to spread and move Qi and Blood, as well as to resolve or dissolve Dampness.

RESEARCHING TCH TO COMBAT CANCER AND CANCER-TREATMENT PAIN

At the time of writing, research is being conducted into Traditional Chinese Herbs (TCH), in the form of formulas, single herbs, or chemical constituents extracted from TCH, in combination with conventional therapies to not only reduce pain from cancer and cancer treatment, but also to keep cancer cells from growing and spreading.

For example, the herb salvia miltiorrhiza bunge (*dan shen*) not only activates Blood circulation and removes Blood stagnation, it also reduces swelling in *toxic sores* (skin lesions that can appear as a side effect of chemotherapy or radiotherapy). A number of studies have shown that some active chemical compounds in *dan shen* have several anti-cancer effects, including preventing or slowing cancer cell growth and production; triggering cancer cell death (*apoptosis*), and hindering the spread of cancer cells to other parts of the body. There's no harm in seeking a consultation with a TCM practitioner for more information or even asking your doctor about their thoughts on this topic. I don't intend to put anyone on the spot, but when it comes to the health of my patients, no stone goes unturned.

According to the Memorial Sloan Kettering Cancer Center, acupuncture increases local blood circulation. The related increase in the availability of oxygen and nutrients to the tissues stimulates healing of surrounding local structures, as well as removing metabolic waste and potentially repairing local nerves.

Increasing appetite

Of course, someone fighting cancer needs to eat to help them keep up their strength throughout the battle. But if a patient has no desire or interest in eating, they can find this necessity difficult to accomplish. Mary felt no hunger, and she didn't find eating appealing at all. She knew she should eat, but her pain and fatigue made it nearly impossible for her to cook (as the family meal preparer), let alone eat.

Based on TCM's Five Elements theory, appetite is associated with the Earth Element (Spleen and Stomach). In the Five Elements relationship cycle, Fire (Heart and Small Intestine, Pericardium, and *San Jiao* [Triple Burner]) supports Earth. Therefore, I selected acupuncture points for Mary on the Spleen, Stomach, Heart, and Pericardium channels to stimulate her appetite.

Among Traditional Chinese Herbs (TCH), ginger (*zingiber officinale,* the ginger plant itself, and *zingiberis rhizoma,* the underground stem structure of the ginger plant) is a go-to herb for appetite stimulation, as well as nausea and vomiting. I recommended that Mary drink ginger tea two to three times a day for her appetite. Although she didn't report nausea, I advised her to try ginger chews (candy made from ginger) or raw ginger with honey if she did get nauseous.

Turning down heat sensations

Like many cancer patients undergoing treatment, Mary suffered heat sensations that she described as hot flushes that felt like her insides were on fire, as well as sudden sweating, mostly at night. These heat sensations occurred randomly and were severe enough to interrupt her sleep and impact her quality of life.

Although hot flushes and night sweats (HFNS) aren't life-threatening, anyone who has experienced them (including yours truly) can share how disruptive and uncomfortable they can be. Although these symptoms commonly appear during menopause, HFNS also commonly accompanies breast, gynecological, and prostate cancer treatments. For example, more than 80 percent of breast cancer patients who take the medication tamoxifen reported troublesome HFNS, and 50 to 80 percent of prostate cancer patients experience *andropause* (male menopause) that includes HFNS. Some patients experience HFNS so severe that they discontinue treatment, jeopardizing their chances for cancer remission and long-term survival.

TCM theory maintains that Yin deficiency (Yin cold energy is inadequate to balance Yang hot energy) typically causes HFNS, so I applied Mary's acupuncture at points selected to regulate the pores — dispersing heat out of the body — and fortify and nourish Yin. A 2016 systematic review in the *Journal of Cancer Research and Therapeutics* concluded that acupuncture significantly reduces HFNS and improves sleep, irritability, pain, and depression.

Modern modifications of a TCH formula called Great Tonify the Yin Pill (*da bu yin wan*) can be extremely effective for HFNS. As noted above, the Yin is not able to keep the Yang in check, which leads to Heat expressing as HFNS. The main ingredient, Rehmanniae Radix Preparata (*shu di huang*) — the root of the Rehmannia glutinosa plant (see Figure 10-5) — nourishes Yin to quell the Heat, clears Heat to support Yin, and produces Body Fluids to cool and moisten. Testudinis Plastrum (*gui ban*) — a type of tortoise shell, another ingredient in this formula, also nourishes Yin and brings down Fire so Heat does not rise to cause sweating and flushing. Together, these herbs represent a Five Elements relationship strategy (see Chapter 2) to strengthen Water in order to control Fire.

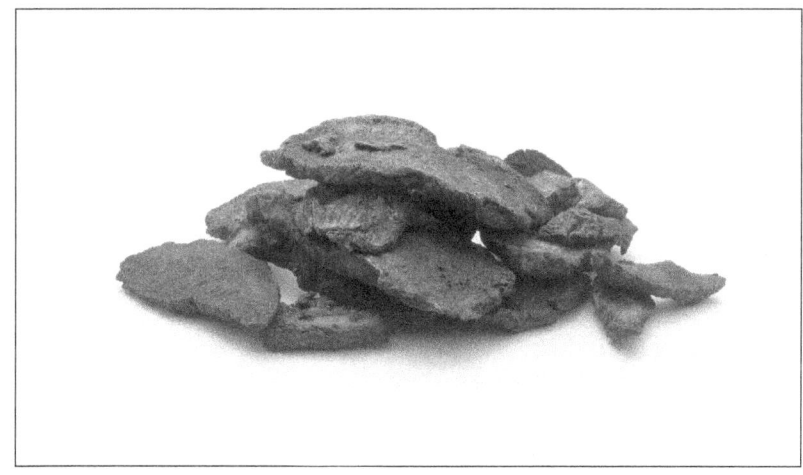

FIGURE 10-5: Rehmannia root is characterized as sweet, warm, moist, and richly tonifying (strengthening).

koosen/Adobe Stock Photos

Easing nausea and vomiting

Thankfully, Mary didn't experience chemotherapy-induced nausea and vomiting (CINV), which is one of the most common and distressing side effects of cancer treatment. It occurs in up to 80 percent of patients and can have a significant impact on a patient's quality of life. According to the National Cancer Institute,

CINV can also result in serious metabolic issues, nutritional deficits, mental and physical deterioration, and withdrawal from cancer treatment.

Researchers have extensively studied acupuncture as a treatment for CINV, as well as garden-variety nausea and vomiting. Acupuncture can help reduce the frequency of CINV and, therefore, reduce the use of medication to control it. One study, "Vitamin B6 Points PC6 Injection During Acupuncture Can Relieve Nausea and Vomiting in Patients With Ovarian Cancer," published in 2009 in the *International Journal of Gynecological Cancer,* determined that acupuncture, combined with an injection of Vitamin B6 at acupuncture point Pericardium-6, provided an effective and safe therapy for CINV.

TIP

Patients can learn acupressure so that they can provide self-care. Applying gentle pressure with a finger, a pencil eraser, or a tablet stylus at Pericardium-6 (about two inches from the wrist on the inner forearm) can help with nausea and vomiting. Acupressure can also help relieve some other common conditions. Please see Chapter 12 for more acupressure points that you can use for yourself or someone else.

A classic Traditional Chinese Herbs (TCH) formula, Six Gentlemen Decoction with Aucklandia and Amomum (*xiang sha liu jun zi tang*), can help patients struggling with CINV. This formula strengthens the Spleen (which makes Qi and Blood), harmonizes the Stomach, regulates Qi, and alleviates pain. It's a digestive tonic that also treats fatigue, tired limbs, and low energy.

POST-TREATMENT CARE

I want to mention what happens to the patient after they complete treatment and enter *remission* (when no cancer is detectable in the body). Most of the current research on the efficacy of TCM for cancer patients focuses on before and during cancer treatment, but very little research examines ongoing therapy in the aftermath of treatment. Many of Western medicine's cancer treatment side effects persist beyond just the time during which the patient actively receives the treatment. The TCM therapies that I used and/or recommended for Mary can certainly apply to cancer survivors because the symptoms that persist, such as nausea, vomiting, fatigue, or pain, haven't changed even if remission has occurred. The same evidence supporting TCM for these symptoms applies because the TCM practitioner is treating the patterns (Dampness, Heat, Yin deficiency, and so on). If it had been available when I was treating Mary, I would have used "Acupuncture and Cancer Survivorship" by Beverley de Valois (2023, Singing Dragon) as a reference.

Closing the Case with Results

Mary reported that she remained nausea-free for the duration of her first round of chemotherapy treatment. Although she continued to feel fatigue, she got her appetite back and had regular bowel movements. After each of her four sessions, she experienced relaxation and pain relief for several days, which allowed her to get better sleep.

Overall, TCM offers cancer patients options for care that can enhance their quality of life during treatment and smooth their road to survival, which can be another challenge — transitioning to life after cancer and dealing with any long-term side effects.

4

The Part of Tens

Chapter **11**

Ten Ways to Eat the TCM Way

S taying healthy in today's fast-paced, short-attention-span, consumption-driven society is *not* easy. And you probably don't have a personal trainer, chef, or food stylist. Like me, you may have tried detox cleanses, diets, a subscription food-delivery service, calorie counting, and fitness/diet apps. Just because I work in the health-care field doesn't mean that I don't have bad habits or indulge in a little too much of a good thing now and then.

My doctors (I have an excellent primary care physician and obstetrician/gynecologist [OB/GYN], among others) give me advice and information. What I do with that advice and information is up to me.

It may be sacrilege to say, but TCM nutrition advice doesn't differ much from general recommendations about healthy food choices and eating habits. The wisdom lies in the application of TCM theory to make choices and form habits that align with nature and your unique constitution.

In this chapter, I share the bits and bobs that TCM theory and my integrative medicine studies revealed to me about healthy eating. You may have heard some of the information in this chapter before, but I hope you consider these recommendations as a gentle reminder to empower you on a path to self-care.

AUTHOR
SAYS

This chapter doesn't provide a comprehensive discussion of TCM nutrition. Instead, these broad brushstrokes touch on food groups and principles to spark your interest in understanding more about how food relates to wellness. TCM nutrition adapts TCM theory to the process of selecting, preparing, and eating your food. You may already practice TCM nutrition without even knowing it!

Eat with Pleasure and Peace

TCM nutrition places a premium on not only what you eat, but also how you eat food. Here are some TCM principles to follow for your meals:

>> **Make colorful meals.** Meals should include foods that reflect the spectrum of colors found in nature and the Five Elements (Earth, Metal, Water, Wood, and Fire; see Chapter 2).

>> **Enjoy foods that smell good, look good, and taste good.** Engage all your senses in the process of preparing and eating food.

>> **Take your time.** Whether alone or in company, don't rush through your meal. Instead, savor the flavors in a relaxed and leisurely way. Not chewing enough or eating too fast can lead to overeating, digestive problems, and surprisingly, an increased risk for malnutrition and dehydration (because you aren't breaking the food down so the nutrients can be properly absorbed).

>> **Prepare your food with attention and intention.** Food can act as medicine, but it can also be filled with love, as every parent or chef can attest.

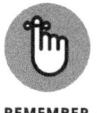

REMEMBER

The word *diet* comes from the Greek word *diaita*, which means "manner of living" or lifestyle. Some people consider food medicine, but the Greeks and Chinese have long understood that food was a component of living well.

Avoid a One-Size-Fits-All Solution

Just as practitioners individualize TCM treatment, they also have to individualize their TCM nutrition recommendations. A TCM practitioner makes food choices according to a person's current condition and situation, medical and dietary history, and constitution.

For instance, insomnia can be caused by worry, pain, depression, medications, caffeine, and so on. In TCM, insomnia can be the result of Excess (too much) Liver

Heat or Deficient (too little) Heart Blood (see Chapter 2). If the imbalance is Excess Liver Heat, the practitioner can recommend foods like bananas or herbs like dandelion root that support and cool the Liver. If the imbalance is Deficient Heart Blood, the practitioner can suggest meat or jujube dates to replenish Heart Blood.

Choose Seasonal and Local Foods

Food in season is at its peak in *Qi* (energy) and nutrients, providing your body with optimum benefits. When you get foods shipped by plane, train, or automobile to reach you, those foods lose their Qi and freshness on the way.

TECHNICAL STUFF

When it comes to produce and fruits, fresh doesn't always mean "not frozen." If produce and fruits are picked at peak ripeness and quickly frozen, they can retain their maximum nutrition and flavor. By contrast, a lot of fresh produce and fruits are picked before they're ripe and then refrigerated for transport to slow deterioration. Research has shown that storage and transport of fruits and vegetables negatively impact their nutrient quality.

Seasonal eating in TCM is directly associated with the Five Elements theory, where each season (spring, summer, late summer, fall, and winter) corresponds to one of the Five Elements (Wood, Fire, Earth, Metal, and Water). In turn, these are linked to the organs and the organ channels (see Chapter 2). For example, Spring is associated with the Wood element, which is linked to the Liver and Gallbladder organs and channels. Therefore, eating foods that are good for the Liver like artichokes, dandelion, and dark leafy greens in the spring will maximize the health of the Liver and Gallbladder. When the season turns to Summer, which is associated with Fire and the Heart-Small Intestine and Pericardium-San Jiao organs and channels, the food choices will shift accordingly.

Select Organic Foods

A lot of research and discussion goes into the effects of the pesticides and chemicals used to grow food and how harmful those chemicals are for humans, animals, plants, ecosystems, habitats, and the planet. When I was growing up, the only *organic* I knew was organic chemistry (and I hated it). So I know that I've ingested toxins and that those toxins impacted my body in some way.

You probably know the same thing about yourself. The good news is that the human body is crazy adaptable and resilient — if you help it out. In addition to choosing seasonal and local foods, as mentioned in the preceding section, choose organic foods to avoid those chemicals.

Organic produce costs more than non-organic, but you don't have to get the organic version of all your produce. When it comes to introducing unwanted chemicals into your body, the worst offenders include produce that have thin skins (such as apples and potatoes) and skins that we eat as part of the package (such as berries, broccoli, and lettuce). Buying produce fresh and rinsing it thoroughly (not just spritzing it with some solution or running water over it for a few seconds) before eating it raw can make a difference. Cooking produce (see the following section) after rinsing it practically eliminates the risk from contaminants. TCM doesn't think cooking food makes it less nutritious. The benefits depend on how you cook your food as noted in the next section.

TIP

If you want to get organic produce that's out of season in your area, frozen is a less expensive way to go than transported fresh (see the previous section on eating local and seasonal). Technology enables producers to freeze fruits and vegetables to keep them as fresh as possible and retain the expected nutrients and flavor. Just check the packaging to confirm the product's organic status, where it was grown and packaged, and the recommended thawing process.

Maximize Foods' Healing Properties

In TCM, cooking methods affect the healing properties of food. There are over 50 different cooking and preparation methods, so this is just a taste. Again, balance is key. To keep it simple, consider the spectrum of methods on the Cold to Hot (Yin to Yang; see Chapter 2) continuum:

- » Cold
  - Raw
  - Pickled
- » Neutral
  - Blanched
  - Steamed
- » Warm
  - Simmered
  - Stewed

- Seared

- Sauteed

» Hot

- Baked

- Roasted

- Fried

- Broiled

- Grilled

Mix up your methods and your foods and note what changes you notice in your body and how you feel.

Consider the Energetic Classification

The therapeutic properties of food are considered much like the therapeutic properties of Traditional Chinese Herbs (TCH) (see Chapter 5). And in the same way that herbs are selected and combined to create a well-balanced formula, foods are selected and combined to create a well-balanced diet. TCM classifies foods in four main areas:

» **Temperature:** The effect that a particular food has on the body. For example, foods classified as hot increase Yang, move up and out, activate *Qi* (energy), and mobilize the defenses. Foods classified as cold counter internal heat, move down and in, and calm the spirit.

» **Flavor:** One of the Five Elements' flavors, associated with specific organs and organ channels: sweet, spicy, sour, bitter, and salty. For example, sweet is the flavor of the Earth element and therefore, sweet foods support the Spleen and Stomach.

» **Organ systems:** Foods that are beneficial to the five organ pairs and their corresponding channels: Lung and Large Intestine, Spleen and Stomach, Heart and Small Intestine (Pericardium and San Jiao [Triple Burner]), Kidney and Urinary Bladder, and Liver and Gallbladder. Chapter 5 covers the therapeutic properties of TCH.

» **Direction:** How the Qi of the food moves within the body: up (ascending), down (descending), sinking (down and in), and floating (up and out).

Eat Food Groups in Sequence

I don't think TCM cornered the market on sequential eating, but it makes sense to eat the densest and richest foods first. The first time I had dinner with my French-California family, the salad came after the main course. Whether you're a carnivore or a vegetarian or somewhere in between, just keep these measures in mind:

>> **Begin a meal by eating high-protein foods.**

Meats and other high-protein foods require the most effort to break down, so you should eat them first to give your body time to start digesting them before digging into your rice or potatoes.

>> **Once you've gotten a headstart with your protein, have something salty like beets or celery in a side dish.**

Salt is Yin, and eating salty flavors stimulates gastric fluids to digest the food that you've already eaten or that you are about to eat. This doesn't mean a bag of potato chips should be a part of every meal. Lightly salting your pasta or potatoes will work just fine.

>> **Greens and non-starchy vegetables come next.**

Eaten with or after your meal, greens and vegetables aid digestion by balancing (or cooling) the heat of the *Stomach Qi* (energy generated to digest your food) that your body needs to process these denser foods.

>> **End your meal with fruits or sweets.**

Sugar can highjack the digestive process because it can cause foods to sit and ferment in the stomach, resulting in gas and bloating. This is why you may have heard, "you can't have that, it will spoil your dinner." Eat fruit or sweets at the end of the meal to avoid diverting your digestive system from breaking down the more nutrient-dense part of your meal.

Drink Liquid in Small Amounts with Meals

It's standard practice in the U.S. to drink a beverage or two — such as water, soda, cocktails, or wine — during or after a meal. At many U.S. restaurants, servers bring you ice water before taking your order. You most likely drink the water while waiting for your food, and the server may refill your water throughout your meal.

In TCM theory, your Stomach, the fireplace that burns the fuel that you provide (in the form of food and liquids), operates best when it's hot. Water, soda, and cocktails are cold or cool. If your Stomach has a weakened or snuffed out fire, the fuel doesn't burn at all, or it burns slowly and incompletely. So you have unprocessed or partially processed food that just takes up space (causing bloating), kind of rots (making your GI tract gassy), doesn't deliver the nutrition that your body needs (leading to all kinds of deficiencies), and either takes its sweet time moving (in the form of constipation) or moves fast and loose (giving you diarrhea) through your body.

TIP

Enjoy a pre-meal drink (cocktail, mocktail, or other cold beverage) with some warm or hot appetizers to balance the cold. Drink small amounts of water during your meal, and use less ice in general so your Stomach (and you) can be happier and healthier.

Know When to Avoid Cold Food and Drink

Avoid drinking or eating anything cold first thing in the morning because, as noted above, the Stomach functions best when it's warm and cold is a shock to its system. Think of your Stomach like yourself in the morning — nice and warm, snug in bed — resting and renewing yourself during sleep. Imagine someone dumping a bucket of cold water on your head. That's what you do to your Stomach when you have yogurt, milk, juice, or a smoothie before you eat anything else. If you think a cold bucket of water as a wake-up call is a great way to start your day, you can ignore this advice.

However, if you think the water-bucket wake-up is a miserable thing to do to someone every day, then maybe start your morning with a cup of warm or hot water. Personally, I have two cups of *Yin-Yang water* each morning before anything else. Follow these steps to make this exotic-sounding concoction:

1. **Measure a 1/2 cup of cold (Yin) water from your fridge or faucet into a mug or coffee cup.**

    The half cup is half of whatever you choose to drink from, and cold is whatever you think is cold.

2. **Boil 1/2 cup water.**

3. **Pour the hot/boiling (Yang) water into the container that holds the Yin water from Step 1.**

4. **Drink the combined water immediately.**

   Drink the Yin-Yang water while it's Goldilocks-approved: just right (meaning what feels warm to you).

The gentle jostle of the Yin-Yang water prepares my stomach to receive, process, and distribute whatever I decide goes in next.

Discover Foods that Best Suit You

I can't detail all the TCM properties of different foods (and drinks) in this chapter. But I can provide a little guidance about categories for food groups and familiar ingredients that you can find at your farmers market or grocery store, grow in your garden, or fish or hunt in the wild. For more information about the TCM properties mentioned in this section, see Chapter 2.

REMEMBER

When TCM theory was being developed, many foods we have today didn't exist, like Twinkies, hot dogs, or pluots (plum-apricots). Applying any TCM theory to your diet requires common sense and adaptation. What's most important is to do what you're willing and able to do.

Whole grains

Here are the TCM properties of whole grains, which make up the largest part of the daily diet in many cultures:

>> **Temperature:** Generally warm, neutral, or cool

>> **Flavor:** Sweet

>> **Organs affected:** Spleen and Stomach

According to Western nutrition, whole grains are:

>> Packed with nutrients and fiber

>> Linked to reduced risk of colorectal cancer, heart disease, and Type-2 diabetes

Whole-grain foods include barley, oats, quinoa, rice, rye, and wheat.

Vegetables

In TCM theory, vegetables cover the full range of temperatures, flavors, and organ systems (Lung, Spleen, Heart, and so on) — making them the perfect complement to whole grains (see the preceding section).

According to Western nutrition, vegetables:

>> Are naturally low in fat and calories

>> Contain many nutrients, such as potassium, dietary fiber, folate, and vitamins A and C

>> May lower your risk for heart disease and certain cancers

Vegetables include asparagus, bell peppers, broccoli, carrots, celery, corn, cucumbers, eggplants, garlic, ginger, green beans, green onions (scallions), kale, lettuce, mushrooms, onions, potatoes, pumpkins, tomatoes, and zucchini.

Animal and plant proteins

TCM theory says that proteins have the following properties:

>> **Temperature:** Warm to hot

>> **Flavor:** Generally sweet

>> **Organs affected:** Depends on individual constitution; can be any organ

>> **Benefits:** Replenish energy, especially in recovery from childbirth, surgery, or physical exertion

>> **When and where to eat:** In winter or cold climates because their thermal nature (temperature) is warming

Western nutrition has the following to say about proteins:

>> Exist in every part of your body — muscle, bone, skin, hair, organs, tissue

>> Fuel energy production

>> Carry oxygen throughout your system

>> Help create antibodies against infection

>> Support making and maintaining healthy cells

Animal proteins can come from beef, chicken, lamb, pork, rabbit, turkey, and venison. You can get plant proteins from sources such as beans, lentils, tempeh, and tofu.

AUTHOR SAYS

In both TCM and Western medicine, research indicates that too much animal protein leads to a host of health problems.

Fish and shellfish

TCM properties vary, depending on whether you're talking about freshwater or saltwater animals. Freshwater fish have the following attributes:

>> **Temperature:** Typically neutral to warm

>> **Flavor:** Sweet or salty

>> **Organs affected:** Spleen, Stomach, and Kidney channels

>> **Benefits:** Strengthen Qi, Blood, and Yang

Saltwater fish and shellfish have these traits:

>> **Temperature:** Cool to cold

>> **Flavor:** Generally salty

>> **Organs affected:** Liver and Kidney channels

>> **Benefits:** Nourish Yin

Western nutrition takes the following view of fish and shellfish:

>> High in protein and unsaturated fats

>> Low in calories, saturated fats, and cholesterol

>> Rich in minerals such as potassium, zinc, iron, and selenium

Fish and shellfish include clams, crabs, lobsters, mackerel, mussels, octopuses, oysters, salmon, sardines, scallops, shrimps (prawn), trout, and tuna.

WARNING

Beware of mercury in seafood and consider how and where your seafood is caught. The National Resources Defense Council has a Smart Seafood and Sustainable Fish Buying Guide (www.nrdc.org/stories/smart-seafood-buying-guide) as well as a downloadable Mercury in Fish reference (www.nrdc.org/sites/default/files/walletcard.pdf).

Fruits

The TCM properties of fruits include:

>> **Temperature:** Generally cool to cold; but some types are neutral and warm

>> **Flavor:** Sweet, sour, or bitter in flavor

>> **When/where to eat:** Warm or hot seasons and climates; avoid in winter

>> **Benefits:** Replenish and preserve Body Fluid to moisten and nourish

Western nutrition describes the following traits for most fruits:

>> Low in fat, sodium, and calories

>> The source of many necessary nutrients, including vitamin C, folate, and potassium

Types of fruits include apples, avocados, bananas, blackberries, blueberries, cherries, figs, grapes, grapefruit, lemons and limes, mangoes, oranges, peaches, pears, pineapples, raspberries, strawberries, and watermelons.

SUPPORTING WEIGHT LOSS AND MANAGEMENT

In my experience with patients, TCM has an approach to weight loss and weight management not much different from Western medicine in that it seeks to reduce appetite, increase activity, and support healthy choices. What's off the table when using TCM is surgery; acupuncture is as invasive as TCM treatments get.

The NADA protocol (discussed in the section "Using the NADA protocol" in Chapter 8) and scalp acupuncture (see Chapter 4) can help lower a patient's craving for food. Based on TCM theory, acupuncture on the body can focus on the organ systems involved in digestion to improve the processing of food (see Chapter 2 for more on TCM principles and theory) that's impeding or slowing the digestive process. For people who haven't been active for some time, tai chi and Qigong offer gentle, easy forms of movement that can kickstart a physical routine (see Chapter 5 for more about these TCM movement therapies).

Researchers can't easily collect data to compare TCM treatments for weight loss and management for a variety of reasons, including the fact that TCM treatment is specific

(continued)

(continued)

to each individual. In most research studies, the same exact treatment must be given to each participant, which is contrary to how TCM is administered. So, each participant would be needled in the same way (for example, shallow depth with no stimulation) at the same acupuncture points. However, the data shows that combined therapies — either TCM with Western therapies or combined TCM therapies — yield the best results.

A comprehensive review published in *Obesity Science and Practice* in May 2024 reported that combined TCM therapies produced better results in the short-term (less than six months) than Western medicine, drugs, or lifestyle changes. Another study published in 2022 in *Frontiers in Pharmacology* revealed the potential of a specific TCM herbal formula for weight loss in comparison with liraglutide, an FDA-approved weight loss medication (also known as a GLP-1 injection, it was originally developed for Type-2 diabetes and later approved for weight loss). The study included 1,360 people; roughly half received the herbal therapy and the other half received liraglutide. After 180 days, the TCM herbal formula performed better than liraglutide in body weight (4.5 pounds versus 2.2 pounds) and BMI (1.8 versus 0.9) reduction.

Overall, medical treatments and medications always need better research to understand their safety and effectiveness, but the more researchers study TCM, the better they can design appropriate study methods and identify its benefits and how to use it for those who need it most. It is widely acknowledged by researchers that TCM techniques have fewer side effects and cost less than conventional treatments.

Chapter **12**

Ten (or So) TCM Points for Self-Care

Y ou may feel a little nervous about going to your first acupuncture appointment. (However, you can receive so many health benefits when it's administered by a license practitioner.) In this chapter, I discuss how you yourself can use a similar technique to not only give you some relief from pain and discomfort but also take a Traditional Chinese Medicine (TCM) therapy for a test drive.

Skilled TCM practitioners can use *acupressure,* which involves applying pressure to known acupuncture points, to treat a variety of ailments without the use of needles.

Although it's difficult (and illegal without a proper license) to needle yourself, acupressure works ideally as a self-care tool because you can use it anywhere. All you need are your fingers or, as I often like to use, the eraser end of a pencil or a tablet stylus. Like fingers, these tools are firm but spongy, so they can provide steady but gentle pressure.

Acupressure is also an excellent way to help children and adolescents with nausea, indigestion, or difficulty falling asleep. I've treated children as young as 2. Even though the points are located in different places, some of them overlap in their actions. So, if a point on the hand for sinus congestion doesn't work, you can press a point on the face for the same purpose. Or alternate and combine them. It can even be a game for children to press one spot while you press the other.

WARNING

Using acupressure on these points can't replace medical care or treatment from a licensed TCM practitioner. They may not work for you, but you do have a reasonable chance that they can help calm an upset stomach or reduce the severity of a headache if you use them properly.

You can easily locate the commonly used TCM acupressure points featured in this chapter. For each point, I provide the English-translated name; the organ channel and number; what acupressure to each point does, according to TCM textbooks; and some of my personal observations. I also provide instructions on how to find their approximate locations so that you know where to place your finger.

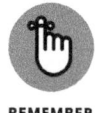

REMEMBER

All of the points that I discuss in this chapter are *bilateral*, meaning on both sides of the body. You can press one side and then the other, or get a partner to help.

Help the Head

This point's name, *Joining Valley*, offers a clue to its location. Large Intestine-4 (LI-4) was probably one of the easiest points for me to memorize and use. LI-4 reminded me of the Vulcan hand sign known to *Star Trek* fans the world over. (I'm a sci-fi geek and proud of it.) The hand sign is accompanied by the phrase, "Live long and prosper," which further solidifies for me the importance of this point. LI-4 is on the back of the hand, in the V shape between the thumb and index finger, as shown in Figure 12-1.

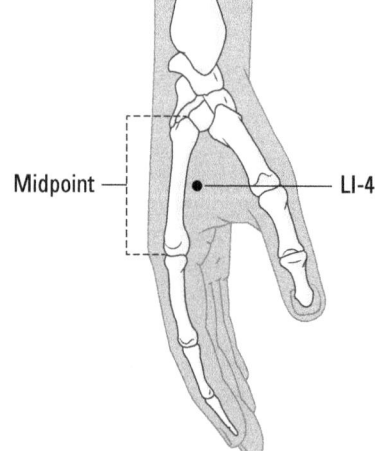

FIGURE 12-1:
Large Intestine-4 (LI-4) is widely used because it treats symptoms affecting the head and sensory organs.

In nearly all the classical TCM texts, LI-4 is the most important point to treat diseases or symptoms affecting the head and the sensory organs (eyes, ears, nose, mouth, or jaw/throat). From headaches and neck aches, to blurry vision and Bell's palsy, to sinus congestion and sweating, LI-4 plays a critical role in many treatments, in combination with other points. I find massaging or pressing LI-4 to be good for taking the edge off a headache and for keeping me chill in both the dentist chair and rush-hour traffic.

WARNING

However, if you're pregnant, consider this acupressure point off limits because when a practitioner uses acupuncture on this point, it stimulates labor. I don't know if acupressure has the same effect as needling, but I wouldn't want to find out.

Open Nasal Passages

Aptly named *Welcome Fragrance*, Large Intestine-20 (LI-20) is the primary local point for nose disorders. It opens the nasal passages, so whether you have a cold or allergies, it can provide temporary relief from a stuffed-up, runny, or itchy nose and slow or stop sneezing and bleeding.

To find LI-20, pinch the bridge of your nose and gently slide your fingers down toward your nostrils until they stop in a little divot just above the opening of the nostrils (see Figure 12-2).

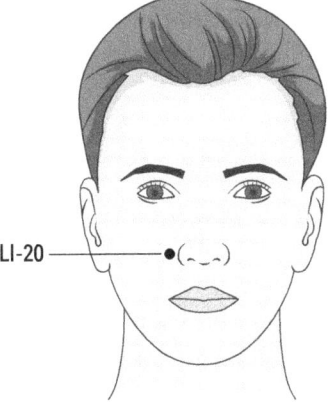

FIGURE 12-2:
As easy to find as the nose on your face, Large Intestine-20 eases stuffiness and congestion.

I suggest this point to patients, family, and friends if they don't have an antihistamine handy.

Walk Three Miles

I can't imagine *not* using *Leg Three Miles*, known as Stomach-36 (ST-36), because using acupressure at this point gives an energy boost for the entire body. It has two interpretations for its name. *Leg* is obviously a reference to its location. How to interpret the *Three Miles* part of the name depends on each practitioner's experience, the TCM diagnosis, and their style of acupuncture (see Chapter 4):

>> According to ancient texts, stimulating this point can enable someone to walk *three* miles beyond their point of exhaustion. Essentially, this point acts like a tonic or a strength enhancer.

>> This point corrects the function of *three* of the Five Element organs introduced in Chapter 4 (Stomach, Spleen, and Kidney), as well as influences *three* sections of the body (upper, middle, and lower).

Regardless of the interpretation, ST-36 is one of the most important points for any issue related to digestion and waste management. In TCM theory, the Stomach breaks down and processes everything that we eat and drink. It sends the good stuff to the rest of the body and sends the bad stuff out to the dump. An upset, unhappy, or malfunctioning stomach creates problems throughout your whole system, so stimulating this point helps the Stomach and its paired organ, the Spleen (see Chapter 2), repair and maintain your digestion.

TIP

Because ST-36 can impact every organ and system in the body, some classic TCM texts recommend needling and applying direct *moxa* (a form of dried mugwort used in *moxibustion,* the burning of mugwort on or near the skin at acupuncture points) regularly to this point for longevity. See Chapters 4 and 5 for more information on acupuncture and moxibustion, respectively.

ST-36 is about 3 to 4-1/2 inches below the bottom of your kneecap, and 1 to 1-1/2 inches to the outside of the *tibia* (the larger of the two lower leg bones that connect your knee and ankle; see Figure 12-3). If you feel downward from your kneecap along the outer edge of the tibia, you may feel a sensitive or tender spot. Massaging the point tends to not only calm my stomach, but also my nervous system.

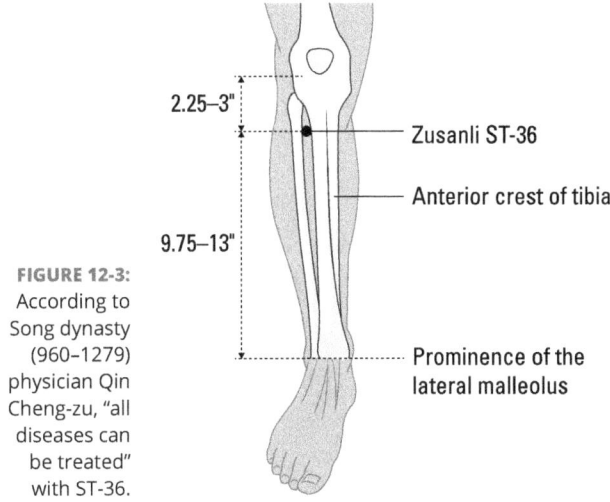

2.25–3"

Zusanli ST-36

Anterior crest of tibia

9.75–13"

FIGURE 12-3:
According to
Song dynasty
(960–1279)
physician Qin
Cheng-zu, "all
diseases can
be treated"
with ST-36.

Prominence of the
lateral malleolus

Benefit the Back

As its English-translated name implies, the *Back Stream (Houxi)* — otherwise known as Small Intestine-3 (SI-3) — acupressure point can benefit the entire spine, but particularly can alleviate back, neck, and *occipital* (back of the head) pain, whether from muscle strain, headache, or joint stiffness. Because of its location, it can also effectively treat finger joint stiffness or pain.

SI-3 is a little tricky to find; it's tucked away in a depression at the base of your pinkie (see Figure 12-4). But with acupressure, you don't have to be as precise as you do in acupuncture. On the pinkie side of your hand, slide from the wrist toward the base of your pinkie. Stop your finger at a bony bump that forms the joint between your hand and pinkie finger. Another way to find SI-3 is to curl your fingers into a loose fist to make your skin fold into creases on the pinkie side. SI-3 is at the edge of the bottom crease.

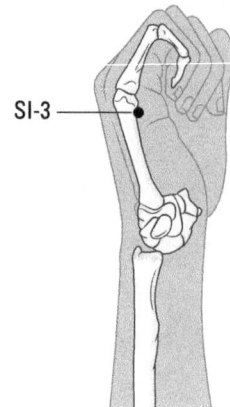

FIGURE 12-4:
Even though
Small Intestine-3
is on the hand, it
is commonly
used for
headaches.

SI-3

Bend the Knee

Traditionally, acupressure at the point *Middle of the Crook (Weizhong),* also known as Urinary Bladder-40 (UB-40), can help treat recurring lumbar pain, which can radiate up the back or affect your ability to straighten your back, making it difficult to bend or stretch your knee.

A fascinating alternative use for Urinary Bladder-40 (UB-40) in classic TCM texts involves treating fevers and heat manifesting on the skin, such as eczema or rashes. But you have to bleed the point to release the heat. To clarify, the process of bleeding a point nowadays (or *bloodletting therapy*) involves nothing more than when you prick a finger to test blood sugar levels — nothing like the days of yore, when people used leeches for bloodletting.

You can find UB-40 in the center of the back of your knee on the popliteal crease, as shown in Figure 12-5. You can find it easy-peasy, but you may perhaps have a little difficulty applying pressure to it yourself. See whether a partner, family member, or friend will massage this point for you, and then you can return the favor.

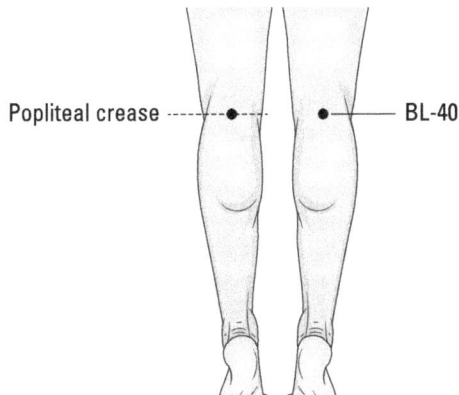

Popliteal crease ----- BL-40

FIGURE 12-5:
Urinary
Bladder-40 can
perform double
duties to help
with low back
pain and
relieve rashes.

Treat Insomnia and Nausea

The point named *Neiguan* or *Inner Gate/Pass* (referred to as Pericardium-6, abbreviated PC-6) predominantly treats diseases in the chest, including heart and lung conditions. PC-6 also plays a primary role in treating a range of emotional disorders — including grief, anxiety, and insomnia — which is no surprise given that the pericardium surrounds the heart (which in TCM is closely associated with one's spirit or emotional soul).

PC-6 is the first point that comes to mind for me (and probably most TCM practitioners) to treat nausea and vomiting, regardless of what's causing the symptoms — motion sickness, pregnancy, food poisoning, chemotherapy, hangover. Colleagues who work in pediatric cancer care show parents how to massage this point on their children's wrists. I've used it myself after late-night celebrations involving fine food and adult beverages.

To find PC-6, turn your hands palm up and make a loose fist. You may see one or both tendons (*palmaris longus* and *flexi carpi radialus*) stand out in the middle of your arm, starting at the crease where your arm meets your hand. If you see only one, you should be able to feel the other one running parallel to it. PC-6 is in the dip between these tendons, two thumb widths (depending on the width of your thumb, of course; about 2–3 inches) from the wrist crease (see Figure 12-6).

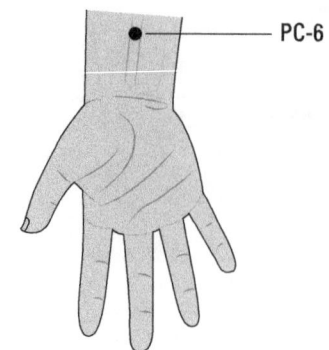

FIGURE 12-6:
Pericardium-6
amazes me
regularly with its
calming effect for
sleep and
digestion.

Alleviate an Ache Up Front

If you get headaches on your forehead, *Yangbai* or *Yang White* is the point for you. Whether it's from sinus congestion, tension, or eye strain, Gallbladder-14 (GB-14) may help ward off the need for an aspirin tablet. This point sits about 1 to 1-1/2 inches above the center of each eyebrow, as shown in Figure 12-7.

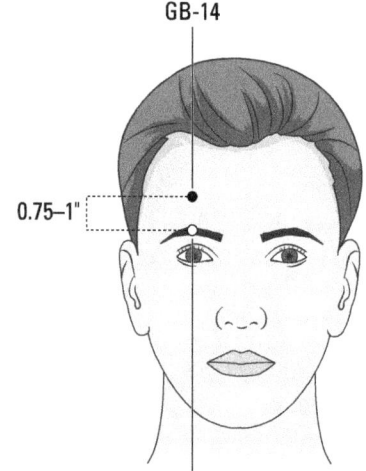

GB-14

0.75–1"

FIGURE 12-7:
Gallbladder-14
is one of my
favorite headache
points.

Stay Centered

Someone could probably write a book about just this point, known as the *Sea of Qi* (*Qihai*) or Conception Vessel-6 (REN-6). Its location in the center of the body, where just about everything happens (eating, processing, reproducing, and so on), indicates the abundance of its applications. REN-6 plays a pivotal role in almost any treatment, as well as in Chinese martial arts and Qigong practice, because your body produces and stores the deepest energies in this area.

In TCM theory, REN-6 can activate the energy that you inherited from your parents and ancestors to support the energy that you make and replenish through nourishment and healthy living (see Figure 12-8). Although using acupressure at this point can provide some relief for a tummy ache, it may feel a bit odd to just press the point, which you can find about 2 to 3 inches directly below your belly button. I prefer to massage the entire area around the belly button to strengthen and/or soothe my entire system. I also think acupuncture with or without moxibustion (see Chapters 4 and 5) is more effective in tapping the benefits of this point.

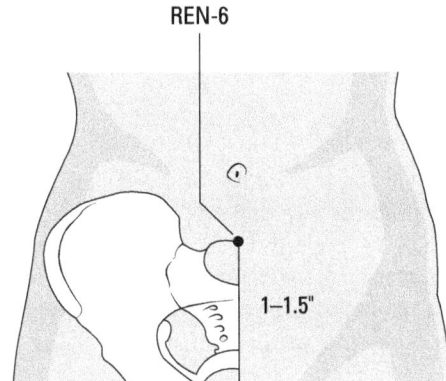

FIGURE 12-8:
REN-6 is an abundant source of Qi (energy) as its name, *Sea of Qi*, implies.

Calm the System

The *Yellow Emperor's Inner Canon* (see Chapter 4), a text from around 2600 BCE, first mentions the *Yintang* (abbreviated as EX-HN-3 for Extra Head and Neck number 3) pressure point, known in many traditional cultures as the third eye or the *Hall of Impression*. TCM practitioners use *Yintang* to calm the system for everything from insomnia and anxiety to hypertension and headache (see Figure 12-9). When my nieces and godchildren were babies and toddlers, I would stroke this point on them to lull them to sleep so successfully that I nicknamed myself Queen Comforter.

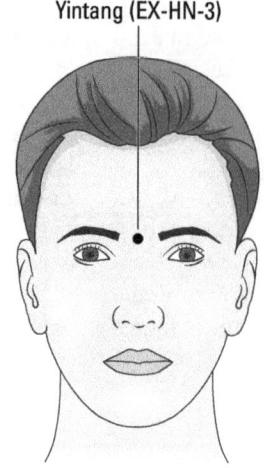

Yintang (EX-HN-3)

FIGURE 12-9:
Yintang may be familiar to yoga practitioners as the third-eye chakra.

Loosen the Neck

If you spend a lot of time staring at a computer screen and bent over a keyboard, or sitting for a long commute in a car or train, the point *Stiff Neck*, or *Luozhen* (abbreviated as EX-UE-14 or EX-UE-8, depending on the textbook, which stands for Extra Upper Extremity point number 14 or 8), can help loosen things up. Pressure to this point can help lessen *acute* (sudden or short-term) neck pain, and you can use it for relief as soon as the pain starts.

Located on the back of the hand, *Luozhen* is in a depression between the second (index finger) and third (middle finger) knuckles, as shown in Figure 12-10.

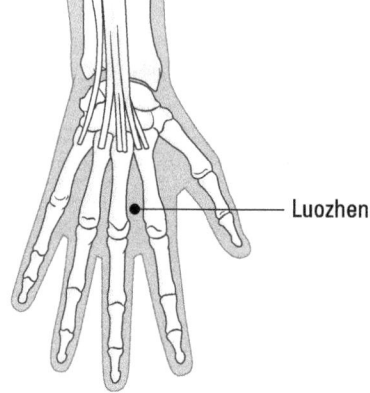

Luozhen

FIGURE 12-10:
Pressing *Luozhen* while gently moving your neck tends to alleviate a stiff neck right away.

Apply Ear Seeds

As discussed in Chapter 4, TCM practitioners use *auricular* (ear) acupuncture around the world. The ear (front and back) provides a miniature replica of the body, so applying acupuncture to specific points on the ear can have the same effect as body acupuncture. I perform ear acupuncture in my practice, but I also apply *ear seeds* (see the next paragraph) at the end of a treatment as needed to let my patients take the treatment home for a while — portable acupressure.

Ear seeds are typically acacia seeds affixed in the center of a very small adhesive patch. These days, other materials are used, such as ceramic beads, tiny magnets, and gold beads. You can apply these patches in different places on the surface of the ear. I tell my patients to massage the patches whenever they think of it, but generally, you massage them two or three times a day to activate them. There's no disadvantage to massaging them more frequently. If you'd rather not use seeds, you can use a cotton swab to massage ear points.

WARNING

Ear seeds usually fall off after three to five days. Please remove them if they stay on longer because bacteria can build up under the patch (like under a bandage). While unlikely for such a small area, keeping the patch on too long could cause a rash or infection.

You can find many ear seed kits online, but even if you don't get yourself a kit, I do recommend that you massage your ears regularly — with or without ear seeds. You can essentially give yourself a full-body massage.

Chapter **13**

Ten (or So) Products for Your Medicine Cabinet

n Western medicine, medications that you can purchase at your local pharmacy or grocery store without a prescription are known as *over-the-counter* (OTC) medicines. Unfortunately, the Traditional Chinese Medicine (TCM) equivalent of OTC medicines is known within the TCM community as *patent medicines,* which leaves me with the bitter aftertaste of the bogus cure-alls that once used that term. Personally, I want to call them TCM OTC medicines, but that's a mouthful. So I go with *TCM medicinals.*

Most TCM medicinals follow a traditional TCM recipe closely, but you can no longer find some ingredients, and the U.S. Food and Drug Administration considers other ingredients unsafe for consumption. Over the centuries, practitioners have made modifications — up to today — while they improve these medicinals for their patients, sort of like culinary chefs adapting classic recipes to elevate diners' experiences.

In this chapter, I give you treatment options for one or more TCM medicinals or supplements to treat 10 common ailments. I picked these treatments up from my integrated medicine studies and personal experience. I recommend these products to my patients and have them in my own medicine cabinet, as well.

I provide the traditional name, its English translation (if available), and any name variations. The name variation indicates some modification to the original formula based on each company's herbal experts. TCM practitioners and herbalists are increasingly mixing and matching Western and Eastern herbs based on availability (or lack thereof), compatibility, and cost. For example, it's cheaper to use herbs grown in the U.S. than to get them from China. In addition, new research and extraction techniques have made it easier to produce TCM medicinals in other forms of administration, such as liquid instead of the traditional herbal powders or pills.

I also include what I use the product for, or the most common signs and symptoms associated with its use, and when *not* to use it.

WARNING

STAYING SHARP IN CHOOSING AND USING TCM MEDICINALS

Although different manufacturers use the same name for a medicinal, each manufacturer may modify the contents of their particular offering. Most of the modifications aren't significant, but I note where it matters. If you need assistance on how to choose TCM medicinals, see the individual entries in this chapter.

Some of the formulas and supplements that I discuss in this chapter have a children's version that comes in liquid form. Please consult a TCM practitioner before giving any of these medicinals to your child because they are smaller than an adult (usually) and recommended dosing is geared toward adults. In addition, a TCM practitioner is most qualified to determine if the formula is appropriate for your child's condition.

I discuss traditional uses or functions for TCM medicinals in this chapter. The U.S. Food and Drug Administration (FDA) doesn't evaluate them, and these products are *not* intended to diagnose, treat, cure, or prevent any disease or condition. If you want to start using one or more of these medicinals, consult a TCM practitioner because that practitioner can guide you in which of these products can best help alleviate the symptoms you are experiencing.

Also, don't use these TCM medicinals and supplements over the long term or frequently. They can help ease discomfort and facilitate the healing of acute (immediate or short-term) conditions. If you have symptoms that don't respond to these TCM medicinals (or any other supplement or medicine, for that matter) or require you to take them frequently for some relief, you have something else going on that requires further examination and evaluation by a medical professional.

I never recommend to anyone a TCM medicinal or supplement that I haven't used myself. I also advise you to talk to your primary care physician before you introduce a new TCM medicinal or supplement into your health-care regimen. Please see Chapter 14 for well-documented herb-drug interactions.

Lastly, always read the labels or check the contents of anything that you put in your body. When in doubt, leave it out.

Stop a Cold in Its Tracks

In my experience, timing is everything — even when a cold starts creeping in. I take Yin Qiao (Chiao) San at the first sign of a cold or flu (usually a sore throat), and nine times out of ten, I can keep the cold from actually becoming a cold. Here are the stats on this medicinal:

>> **Name variation:** Yin Qiao Jin

>> **What it treats:** Common cold or flu (stops progression, shortens duration, or lessens severity of symptoms); sore throat, fever, and chills (with sore throat predominant); cough; stuffy nose caused by yellow mucus

>> **Caution:** Avoid if you're pregnant because introducing any new substance at this time, without proper consultation, can have unintended harmful effects

Harmonize Your Tummy

I don't know about you, but when my stomach is unhappy, so am I. The TCM medicinal Bao He Wan (Preserve Harmony Pill) is aptly named, keeping your stomach calm so you can carry on. However, in my mind, you should take Bao He Wan as prescribed, not without guidance, because its traditional use is for food poisoning or after eating and drinking too much. So the following sections offer three alternatives to Bao He Wan that I recommend readily (and carry in my purse).

Kang Ning Wan

Kang Ning Wan, similar to Bao He Wan, provides relief from almost any digestive issue. Here are the details on this medicinal:

>> **English translation:** Curing (Culing) Pills

>> **Name variations:** Bao Ji Wan or Po Chai Pills

>> **What it treats:** This medicinal has several uses. It can treat

- Digestive issues

- Symptoms of a hangover, such as any of the issues listed below, as well as mild headache and a feeling of "brain fog" (This is not a traditional use but is based on my personal experience and the experience of others)

- Low appetite

- Feeling stuffed; bloating and/or distension

- Gas and indigestion

- Gurgling/uneasy stomach

- Nausea and vomiting

- Heartburn/acid reflux

>> **Caution:** Avoid using this medicinal if you're pregnant because introducing any new substance at this time, without proper consultation, can have unintended harmful effects; or if you have chronic or recurring gastrointestinal conditions/issues because this formula is not intended for long-term use

Papaya

Papaya (whether fresh or as an enzyme tablet) has the following characteristics:

>> **What it treats:** Bloating, indigestion, or stomach discomfort.

>> **Caution:** Avoid if you're pregnant because unripe (green skin) papaya contains latex, which triggers contractions or early labor. It's unclear whether the enzyme is a safe option during pregnancy. Please check with your doctor.

TIP

Use fresh papaya if you can because this is its natural state (that is, not processed) and it tastes good (in my opinion); otherwise, you can find papaya enzyme tablets available at most natural grocery stores or online. You'll find dosage instructions for the enzyme tablets on the bottle. The amount of fresh papaya depends on each person. A few slices do the trick for me, and my mother ate a few slices every morning (if available) as a preventative measure.

Ease the Exit

What leaves your body is just as important as what you put in it. Regularly emptying the trash — so to speak — keeps your digestion and the rest of your body in good shape. For the occasional bout of constipation, Run Chang Wan can help your body move out waste:

>> **English translation:** Moisten the Intestines Pill

>> **What it treats:** Constipation (particularly for children, elders, or people who have a weak constitution because it's quite gentle), dry stools, infrequent bowel movements, and difficulty with bowel movement

>> **Caution:** Avoid if you're pregnant because introducing any new substance at this time, without proper consultation, can have unintended harmful effects

WARNING

If the formula variation contains the herb Da Huang (rhubarb root and rhizome), it will be more forceful and may clear out too much. Ask a TCM practitioner for more information.

Relieve a Headache

Everyone experiences a headache now and then. And it's wise to keep something in the cabinet to help when one hits. Common OTC medications — ibuprofen, acetaminophen, or aspirin — are used for headaches. They can also ease muscle aches, reduce fever, or help prevent a heart attack. However, long-term use of these can damage your liver, kidneys, or stomach.

The following items don't impact your organs, so I use them as an alternative, depending upon the source of the headache. For example, if I have a headache with a fever, I take acetaminophen. If I have a headache with body aches, I use ibuprofen or arnica (see below). If I have any other kind of headache (tension, eye strain, late-night out), I use the formula below.

Chuan Xiong Cha Tiao Wan

I recommend the TCM medicinal Chuan Xiong Cha Tiao Wan (also called its short-ened name, Chuan Xiong Wan) as an alternative to OTC headache medications:

- **English translation:** *Ligusticum striatum* (the scientific name of the plant); Powder to Be Taken with Green Tea

- **Name variations:** Head-Q, Ligusticum Teapills

- **What it treats:** Acute or occasional headache; pain in any part of the head caused by stress, tension, anxiety, cold/flu, sinuses, or menstruation

WARNING

Avoid taking this medicinal if you're pregnant because introducing any new sub-stance at this time, without proper consultation, can have unintended harm-ful effects.

Arnica

Arnica, as a gel, cream, or pill that you can use topically or orally, provides pain relief:

- **What it treats:** Topical: aches, pains, sprains, strains, bumps, or bruises; oral: headaches and body aches

WARNING

For the topical version, avoid using it on open cuts/wounds or irritated, inflamed skin because it can further irritate the wound or skin.

WARNING

Migraines are another category of headache, and these require tailored TCH formulas rather than a standard TCM medicinal.

Avoid a Runny Nose

I used to have terrible hay fever growing up. I dreaded three out of four seasons, strong winds, and open spaces that contained wildflowers and grass. I wish I had known about the following three TCM medicinals, which treat sinus congestion and discharge because of cold, flu, allergy, or infection.

Which medicinal to choose depends on the cause (infection, virus, or allergy) and the symptoms. Consult a TCM practitioner to help you make the best choice:

>> **Pei (Bi) Min Kan Wan:** Nasal Pills (English translation)

>> **Cang Er Zi San (Wan):** Upper Chamber Teapills (English translation); also called Xanthium Powder

>> **Bi Yan Pian:** Nose Inflammation Tablets (English translation)

All three of these medicinals have common uses and cautions:

>> **Name variations:** Magnolia (or Pueraria) Clear Sinus, Nasal Caps 2

>> **What they treat:** Sinus congestion (stuffy nose), discharge (clear and thin, or thick and yellowish), sneezing, and itchy nose and/or eyes

WARNING

Avoid if you're pregnant because introducing any new substance at this time, without proper consultation, can have unintended harmful effects. Also, this product may overly dry out your nasal passages.

Boost Your Immunity

Even though your immune system relies on nutrients such as vitamins and minerals and properly functioning biological systems, the classic TCM medicinal Yu Ping Feng San tells you what it does in its translated name — Jade Windscreen Powder. It shields you from external pathogens that cause colds or allergic reactions:

TIP

>> **Name variations:** Xanthium Relieve Surface, Immune +

You can find plenty of adaptations available, but in my experience, forms of this medicinal that use the traditional name are most effective, according to my patients who take them

>> **What it treats:** Boosts the immune system for recurring or chronic colds, allergies, and asthma; seasonal allergies, such as hay fever, sinus congestion

I haven't encountered or read about any negative effects from this medicinal, so I have no cautions to give.

Stop Bleeding

If you've ever nicked yourself in the kitchen, fallen on a hike or off a bike, or sparred too hard in martial arts or boxing, you've experienced cuts and scrapes. Cleaning and applying pressure are standard procedures, but you can also help stop the bleeding by applying Yunnan Baiyao:

>> **English translation:** White Medicine of Yunnan

>> **What it treats:** Bleeding, pain, and healing/recovery from injury/surgery; cuts, bruises, and wounds

WARNING

Avoid taking this medicinal if you're pregnant because introducing any new substance at this time, without proper consultation, can have unintended harmful effects. Also, avoid it if you have heart or bleeding conditions because it contains an organic compound (an alkaloid) that can potentially harm anyone with compromised heart function.

Stop Coughing

Although the medicinal Nin Jiom Pei Pa Koa is a cough suppressant, it can also help treat a sore or dry throat from a cold or overuse:

>> **English translation:** Honey and *Loquat* (a type of fruit) Syrup.

Although the name includes the word *syrup,* you can also find it available as lozenges in different flavors.

>> **What it treats:** Coughing; sore or dry throat.

I haven't encountered any cautions in taking this medicinal (except maybe using more syrup or lozenges than necessary because they taste good).

Alleviate Aches and Pains

The three *liniments* (herbs in oil) that I discuss in this section can treat pain caused by a variety of conditions, from injury to overuse to arthritis. Personally, I alternate them with CBD (cannabidiol, a compound in cannabis) balms for my osteoarthritis. Here are my go-to topical pain treatments (for aches, pains, sprains, strains, bumps, or bruises):

>> Dr. Shir's Liniment

>> Zheng Gu Shui

>> Po Sum On Medicated Oil

>> Arnica (see above)

WARNING

Avoid using any of these liniments on open cuts or wounds, or irritated, inflamed skin, because they can further irritate the wound or skin.

Get Some Sleep

I have nights when I can't turn my brain off, and it takes a while to fall asleep. If I'm not asleep within 30 minutes, I know my Circadian rhythm is off, and I'm probably going to have a rough night. This TCM medicinal, An Mian (Mien) Pian, helps turn out my lights (metaphorically) on those occasions:

What it treats: Occasional insomnia, difficulty falling and/or staying asleep.

Know How to Choose TCM Medicinals

Like Western medicine OTC treatments, you can find TCM medicinals in pharmacies and supermarkets, as well as online. Despite the convenience and cost-effectiveness of online shopping, I caution my patients about purchasing TCM medicinals and supplements from unfamiliar sources or from a website that can't verify the legitimacy of its products.

The National Institutes of Health (NIH), Office of Dietary Supplements (ODS) is responsible for coordinating and distributing scientific research on dietary supplements across the NIH and other federal agencies, such as the Food and Drug Administration (FDA). Before buying any medications, get familiar with three terms for nutritional products sold in the U.S.:

>> **Dietary supplements:** This category includes (or is a combination of) vitamins, minerals, herbs and their extracts, amino acids, and enzymes. You must ingest them, like they're part of your diet. Lotions or creams that you apply to your skin, known as *topicals,* don't count as dietary supplements because they are not nutritional products that you consume.

>> **Herbal medicines:** These products are *botanicals* (meaning they are made from plants or parts of plants), some of which are also dietary supplements. Most, but not all, TCM medicinals fall under this definition.

>> **Nutraceuticals:** Also called *functional food,* the name *nutraceuticals* (a combination of "nutrition" and "pharmaceutical") refers to the nutrients derived from food sources that may have some health benefits. In the simplest terms, they are substances like ginseng, *Echinacea,* or omega-3 fatty acids that have proven or potential therapeutic effects.

The rapid rise of dietary supplements occurred after the U.S. Congress passed the Dietary Supplement Health and Education Act (DSHEA) of 1994, which basically removed the FDA's authority to regulate dietary supplements. The FDA doesn't test or approve these products for safety and effectiveness. Manufacturers can put dietary supplements on the market without the FDA even knowing about it.

So, if no one's checking, how confident can I (or you) be about what's in these products, how they're made and packaged, how they get transported or delivered, whether the recommended dose is the actual effective dose, and what they'll do after I (or you) take them?

Because I can't answer these questions definitively, I make it a point to get my Sherlock Holmes hat on and investigate the product myself, which I do for just about anything that I purchase with my hard-earned cash — and especially for something that's going into my body.

The following list shows my process for deciding whether to use a medicinal. Follow these steps to do your own investigation:

1. **Look up the manufacturer's information.**

   - Get their registration or license (through the secretary of state, city business license department, and so on): Is it active, suspended, or not found?

   - Online reviews from customers.

   - Social media presence (whether they have accounts and the level of activity on those accounts).

   - Rating/review with the Better Business Bureau (but not every business is rated by them).

2. **Verify their physical address (and visit, if they're local).**

3. **Find their phone number and call to talk to a representative to ask about their manufacturing process and where their materials come from.** Ask anything that you want to know that will help you evaluate their product.

4. **Check out their website to see what they say about themselves and their products.**

5. **Check to see whether they belong to an industry or trade association, and/or if they are Good Manufacturing Practices (GMP)-certified.**

   For dietary supplements, these associations include the American Herbal Products Association (AHPA), the Consumer Healthcare Products Association (CHPA), the Council for Responsible Nutrition (CRN), and the United Natural Products Alliance (UNPA). GMP guidelines were first established by the World Health Organization in 1968 and updated in 1991. These guidelines are legal requirements in more than 100 countries and enforced by agencies like the FDA in the U.S. and the European Medicines Agency. Certification indicates the company has demonstrated through an audit that they follow GMP.

6. **Ask for advice.**

   Trusted colleagues, family, friends, and medical professionals may be able to give you advice on products that they've used.

7. **Look at trusted consumer-oriented review sources.**

   Websites such as Consumer Reports (www.consumerreports.org) or the Environmental Working Group (www.ewg.org) can help you get the scoop on a particular manufacturer.

Chapter **14**

Treating Ten Health Issues with Drugs and Herbs

don't think of myself as an herbalist, but I play one on TV (just kidding). However, I'm probably more of an herbalist than a layperson. I'm definitely not a pharmacologist. But I don't have to be one to understand that very bad things can happen if you mix substances that don't play well together.

Although I have a particular affinity and preference for herbs used in Traditional Chinese Medicine (TCM), I also appreciate the speed with which an antibiotic can knock out an infection. I guess what I'm trying to say is that, from my perspective, everything has a time and place.

A 2015 National Health Interview Survey (from the U.S. Centers for Disease Control and Prevention) reported that more than one-third (38–42 percent) of U.S. adults used herbal medicines with either prescription drugs or over-the-counter (OTC) medications. So, you can combine drugs and herbal remedies safely (and many people do just that).

In this chapter, I'd like to present drugs and herbs — botanicals and Traditional Chinese Herbs (TCH) — in ten categories of therapeutic action (what they are commonly used to treat). On the one hand, medicines (in this chapter, I'm referring to drugs and herbs collectively) with similar effects may enable you to take less of one (a drug) and more of the other (an herb). On the other hand, taking medicines with the same effects, regardless of the amount, can also be toxic to you. How medicines interact with each other and with your body determines which hand you'll be dealing with. Therefore, this chapter also provides a general overview of drug interactions.

REMEMBER

Consult medical professionals who know about drug and herb interactions. Herbs, drugs, and herb-drug interactions are required curriculum for licensed TCM practitioners and practitioners who obtain national certification in Chinese Herbology (see Chapter 3, Accessing TCM). Some medical doctors may also receive training on herbs, their uses, and their interactions with drugs. The lists in this chapter give you a heads-up about what to look out for so that you can ask the right questions and receive the right treatment.

Your primary care physician and TCM practitioner should always consider your current medications, supplements, diet, and health condition(s) before they recommend any new drugs, herbs, or supplements.

Understanding Basic Drug Interactions

When it comes to how drugs can interact with herbs, other drugs, supplements, or even food, many complex biological, chemical, and physiological processes are at work. I promise not to bore you with an organic chemistry lesson, but as a consumer, you need to have some idea of what happens to your body when you take a drug.

How your body absorbs, distributes, metabolizes, and eliminates (ADME) a drug is known as *pharmacokinetics*. After a drug enters your body by mouth or by injection, it moves into your bloodstream by absorption, mainly through your intestinal walls. Then your blood delivers the drug, releasing it to the target organs, tissues, and cells (a process called *distribution*). Your body (usually by using enzymes in your liver) chemically alters and breaks down the drug as a part of *metabolism*. Then, the broken-down drug can leave your body (through *elimination*) — because you don't want it hanging around any longer than necessary.

Five main effects that can occur when a drug interacts with an herb or another drug:

>> **Addition:** You take two drugs that have similar actions, and you can achieve the same effect while using a lower dose of each; considered a *positive effect* because you can achieve the same result with less of each drug, which reduces the chance of adverse reactions and tolerance (*the more you use a drug, the less effective it becomes*).

>> **Synergism:** When you take two drugs with similar properties and achieve a greater therapeutic effect than each alone. However, the combination can also result in a greater adverse reaction. Therefore, synergism can be *positive*, such as more or faster improvement in your condition, or *negative*, such as nausea or upset stomach.

>> **Potentiation:** When one drug enhances or boosts the effect of another drug that can't be effective on its own. However, the combination can also increase the risk of an adverse reaction. Therefore, this combination can have a *positive* or *negative effect* (similar to synergism above).

>> **Antagonism:** You take two drugs and end up with a lesser therapeutic effect (or no effect at all) than if you took each drug individually. In some cases, one drug may negate or block the effect of the other. This is considered a *negative effect* because there is little or no improvement in your condition as the drugs cancel each other out.

>> **Incompatibility:** If you combine two drugs and the number or severity of adverse reactions increases. A *very negative effect,* meaning toxicity is building in your body, that usually occurs when one drug hinders another drug's metabolism and/or elimination.

Any interaction depends on your ADME and careful monitoring and observation of your response by you and your medical professional, whether Western or Eastern. It's my opinion that *synergism* presents the highest risk of drug-herb interactions because it's quite natural to want more of a good thing. But with synergism, over-dosing can be harmful to you and prevent you from getting the effect(s) you need to improve or maintain your health.

So, with this in mind, I've prepared the following sections with medicines (drugs, herbs, and TCH) that have similar therapeutic actions but should be combined with caution (or not at all) because of their potential for overdosing. In some cases, I've included antagonistic interactions. In addition, for the drugs, I have provided brand name examples since brand names may be more familiar than the generic or pharmaceutical name.

Activating the Nervous System

Sympathomimetic drugs, herbs, or other substances mimic the sympathetic nervous system (the fight or flight response) — increasing heart rate and blood pressure, slowing digestion, and maximizing blood flow to the brain and muscles. These drugs range in use from stuffy noses to heart failure. Some common examples of these medicines include:

>> **Drugs:** Epinephrine (Adrenalin), albuterol (ProAir HFA), amphetamine (Adderall), caffeine, cocaine, dopamine (Intropin), isoproterenol (Isuprel), and pseudoephedrine (Sudafed)

>> **Herbs:** Bitter or Seville orange (*Citrus aurantium*)

>> **TCH:** Zhi Shi (Fructus aurantii immaturus), Ma Huang (Herba ephedrae)

WARNING

Combining these medicines can be overstimulating to your nervous system, such as raising your blood pressure too much, making you jittery, or causing insomnia. Antagonistically, these medicines may interfere with antihypertensive (a *class of drugs used to treat high blood pressure*) or antiseizure (a *class of drugs used to prevent or treat seizures*) medications.

Slowing Blood Clot Formation

Anticoagulants are also known as blood thinners because they slow down the blood's clotting process. Practitioners often prescribe these medicines to prevent strokes and heart attacks. Some common examples of these medicines include:

>> **Drugs:** Apixaban (Eliquis), heparin, rivaroxaban (Xarelto), warfarin (Coumadin)

>> **Herbs:** Chamomile (*Matricaria recutita, Chamaemelum nobile*), fenugreek (*Trigonella foenum-graecum*), red clover (*Trifolium pratense*)

>> **TCH:** Dan Shen (Radix salvia miltiorrhizae), Dang Gui (Radix angelicae sinensis), Chuan Xiong (Rhizoma ligustici chuanxiong), Tao Ren (Semen persicae), and Hong Hua (Flos carthami)

WARNING

Combining these medicines can lead to prolonged or excessive bleeding because they may thin your blood too much.

Among anticoagulants, warfarin (Coumadin) is the most troublesome because it requires careful dosing and regular lab testing to avoid serious complications.

I don't recommend any TCH or supplements to patients who are taking warfarin unless I can consult directly with their doctor. And even then, I'm wary.

Averting Blood Clots

Antiplatelet medications prevent platelets in the blood from clumping together. Although platelets act as nature's way of keeping us from bleeding until we're bloodless, too much clumping can create blood clots that can lead to stroke or heart attack. Some common examples of these medicines include:

>> **Drugs:** Aspirin, clopidogrel (Plavix), cilostazol (Pletal), dipyridamole (Persantine), tirofiban (Aggrastat), vorapaxar (Zontivity)

>> **Herbs:** Barberry (*Berberis vulgaris*), garlic (*Allium sativum*), ginger (*Zingiber officinale*), magnolia (*Magnolia officinalis*), turmeric (*Curcuma longa*)

>> **TCH:** Da Suan (Bulbus alli sativi), Dang Gui (Radix angelicae sinensis), Gan Jiang (Rhizoma zingiberis), Hou Po (Cortex magnoliae officinalis), Huang Lian (Rhizoma coptidis), Jiang Huang (Rhizoma curcumae longae), Yu Jin (Radix curcumae)

WARNING

Like anticoagulants, combining these medicines can lead to prolonged or excessive bleeding because they may thin your blood too much.

TECHNICAL STUFF

You may have noticed that *Dang Gui (Radix angelicae sinensis)* appears in both the anticoagulant and antiplatelet sections. Antiplatelet drugs prevent only platelets from forming, while anticoagulants slow the entire process of clot formation. Like many TCH, Dang Gui does not have a single indication. Its properties make it effective for many blood-related conditions such as irregular heartbeat (arrhythmia) and stroke, and therefore, has anticoagulant and antiplatelet effects.

Lowering Blood Pressure

Medical professionals prescribe *diuretics*, also known as *water pills*, to help lower blood pressure by encouraging the kidneys to eliminate more salt and water from the body through urination. Some common examples of these medicines include:

>> **Drugs:** Furosemide (Lasix), hydrochlorothiazide (Esidrix), triamterene (Dyrenium)

» **Herbs:** Dandelion (*Taraxacum officinale*), garlic (*Allium sativum*), ginger (*Zingiber officinale*), parsley (*Petroselinum crispum*)

» **TCH:** Fu Ling (*Poria*), Zhu Ling (*Polyporus*), Che Qian Zi (*Semen plantaginis*), Ze Xie (*Rhizoma alismatis*)

WARNING

Combining these medicines can cause your blood pressure to go too low, leading to dizziness or fainting.

Controlling Blood Sugar

Controlling blood sugar resonates with me personally because I was on the doorstep of Type-2 diabetes for several years before COVID, family deaths, and depression pushed me over the line. Like many Type-2 patients, I take an *antidiabetic* medication to help control my blood sugar. Combined with lifestyle changes such as watching what I eat, exercising, and managing stress, I lowered my *A1C* (a blood test value used to measure your average amount of blood sugar over several months) to prediabetes levels in six months. I want to manage my blood sugar levels by maintaining my lifestyle choices and taking a synergistic approach by lowering my medication and adding TCH for support. Some examples of medicines in this category include:

» **Drugs:** Acarbose (Precose), empagliflozin (Jardiance), glimepiride (Amaryl), metformin (Glucophage), nateglinide (Starlix), sitagliptin (Januvia)

» **Herbs:** Ceylon cinnamon (*Cinnamomum zeylanicum*), fenugreek (*Trigonella foenum-graecum*), ginger (*Zingiber officinale*), ginseng *(Panax ginseng)*, white mulberry (*Morus alba*)

» **TCH pairs:** Zhi Mu (Radix anemarrhenae) and Shi Gao (Gypsum fibrosum), Xuan Shen (Radix scrophulariae) and Cang Zhu (Rhizoma Atractylodis), Shan Yao (Rhizoma Dioscoreae) and Huang Qi (Radix astragali)

TECHNICAL
STUFF

Based on TCM theory and the properties or actions associated with individual herbs, paired herbs can achieve the positive effects of synergism or potentiation while minimizing or eliminating any negative effects. Therefore, individually, these herbs do not have antidiabetic actions.

Stopping Seizures

Antiseizure medications (formerly called antiepileptic or anticonvulsant medications) help to treat and/or prevent seizures caused by temporary, unexpected electrical surges that occur in the brain. Seizures cause more than convulsions; they can also cause confusion and loss of consciousness. (Hence, the change in category name to *antiseizure.*) Some examples of these medicines include:

>> **Drugs:** Cannabidiol (Epidiolex), carbamazepine (Epitol, Tegretol), ethosuximide (Zarontin), gabapentin (Horizant, Gralise, Neurontin), phenobarbital (Solfoton, Luminal), phenytoin (Dilantin, Phenytek)

>> **Herbs:** Black cumin (*Nigella sativa*), cannabis (*Cannabis sativa*), cilantro (*Coriandrum sativum*)

>> **TCH:** Bai Shao (Radix paeoniae alba), Gou Teng (Ramulus uncariae cum uncis), Shi Chang Pu (Rhizoma acori), Tian Ma (Rhizoma gastrodiae)

WARNING

Combining medicines in this category presents the risk of more severe side effects, such as cognitive impairment or even increased seizures from neurotoxicity.

Relieving Depression

Selective serotonin reuptake inhibitors (SSRIs) are the most prescribed class of antidepressants because they usually have fewer and less severe side effects than other classes. In TCM theory, depression results from an imbalanced or unsettled spirit (see Chapter 8). Your *shen* is your emotional and psychological center. When it is balanced and calm, you are content and focused. You sleep, eat, and engage with others well. In short, when your *shen* is balanced, you are mentally healthy. Some examples of medicines in this category include:

>> **Drugs:** Citalopram (Celexa), escitalopram (Lexapro), fluoxetine (Prozac), paroxetine (Paxil, Pexeva), sertraline (Zoloft)

>> **Herbs:** Black cohosh (*Actaea racemosa* or *Cimicifuga racemosa*), chamomile (*Matricaria recutita, Chamaemelum nobile*), chasteberry (*Vitex agnus-castus*), lavender (*Lavandula*), passionflower (*Passiflora incarnata*), saffron (*Crocus sativus*), St. John's wort (*Hypericum perforatum*)

>> **TCH:** Guan Ye Lian Qiao (*Herba hypericum*), He Huan Pi (*Cortex albiziae*), Xiao Mai (*Fructus tritici*)

WARNING

Combining these medicines can lead to toxic levels of serotonin with symptoms ranging from restlessness and seizures to sweating and loss of consciousness. According to the National Center for Complementary and Integrative Health, St. John's wort, in particular, limits the effectiveness of many prescription medications.

Treating Insomnia

Based on the 2020 National Health Interview Survey, approximately 32.3 percent of adults (over age 18) in the U.S. have trouble falling asleep or staying asleep. *Sleeping pills* make people feel drowsy and relaxed to help them with insomnia. OTC sleep aids typically contain an antihistamine such as diphenhydramine (for example, Benadryl). Prescription sleeping pills can come from a different class of medication, such as antidepressants, barbituates, and benzodiazepines.

In TCM, insomnia has a variety of underlying causes linked to specific TCM diagnoses (see Chapter 2 for more on TCM concepts). However, insomnia is often a sign of some kind of *shen* imbalance (see the previous section, "Relieving Depression"). TCHs are selected based on the underlying cause of the *shen* imbalance. Some common examples of medicines in this category include:

>> **Drugs:** TCAs and SSRIs (antidepressants; see "Using One Drug for Multiple Conditions," later in this chapter, and the preceding section); amobarbital and secobarbital (barbiturates); alprazolam, clonazepam, diazepam, lorazepam, temazepam (benzodiazepines); zolpidem and eszopiclone (sedative-hypnotics)

>> **Herbs:** German chamomile (*Matricaria recutita*), lemon balm (*Melissa officinalis*), valerian (*Valerian officinalis*)

>> **TCH:** Bai Jiang Cao (Herba cum radice patriniae), Dan Shen (Radix salvia miltiorrhizae), He Huan Pi (Cortex albiziae), Xiao Mai (Fructus tritici), Suan Zao Ren (Semin zizyphi spinosae), Xie Cao (Radix et rhizome valerianae)

WARNING

It may be obvious to say, but combining these types of medicines can make you sleepy, slow to react, or unconscious.

Loosening Anxiety's Grip

Anxiolytics are drugs that treat anxiety and related conditions. Derived from two ancient Greek words ("anxio" means anxiety and "lytic" means "to loosen"), they are also known as *anti-anxiety* medications. Anxiolytics come from a range of different drug categories, many of which I've already discussed in earlier sections, such as antidepressants.

In TCM, anxiety also stems from a *shen* imbalance. TCHs are selected based on the underlying cause of the *shen* imbalance.

>> **Drugs:** Alprazolam (Xanax), clonazepam (Klonopin), diazepam (Valium), escitalopram (Lexapro), lorazepam (Ativan), paroxetine (Paxil)

>> **Herbs:** German chamomile (*Matricaria recutita*), kava (*Piper methysticum*), lavender (*Lavandula*), lemon balm (*Melissa officinalis*), passionflower (*Passiflora incarnata*), valerian (*Valerian officinalis*)

>> **TCH:** Bai Zi Ren (Semen platycladi), Gui Ban (Plastrum testudinis), Long Gu (Os draconis), Wu Wei Zi (Fructus schisandrae chinensis), Xiao Mai (Fructus tritici), Yu Jin (Radix curcumae)

WARNING

Combining medicines in this category increases the risk of motor and memory impairment, drowsiness, and depression. The drugs in this category are highly addictive and can have very unpleasant withdrawal symptoms such as insomnia, anxiety, and sensory hypersensitivity.

Using One Drug for Multiple Conditions

Tricyclic antidepressants (TCAs) are an older class of antidepressants originally used to help manage the symptoms of clinical depression. However, doctors now prescribe them more commonly for other conditions, such as insomnia, anxiety, migraine, and chronic pain. TCAs help to maintain higher levels of serotonin and norepinephrine, which influence mood, attention, and pain. Hence, TCAs can be highly effective for depression and continue to be prescribed for patients who do not respond to first-line treatment (*the initial or preferred treatment option for a specific medical condition*), such as SSRIs (see the previous section, "Relieving Depression").

TECHNICAL
STUFF

Using TCAs for conditions other than the conditions they were originally created to treat is an example of *off-label* or unapproved use. The U.S. Food & Drug Administration (FDA) is the federal authority that approves drugs (not herbs or supplements) to treat human disease and illness. Other types of off-label use include changing the dosage (two pills instead of one) and changing how the drug is administered (e.g., it was approved as a pill, but it is being offered as a liquid). Off-label use is common, but patients should understand what it means and why it is being recommended. For a more thorough explanation, you can visit the

FDA's page on this topic: https://www.fda.gov/patients/learn-about-expanded-access-and-other-treatment-options/understanding-unapproved-use-approved-drugs-label.

Herbs and TCH that have the same action on serotonin and norepinephrine are included in this category. However, not all the TCH may be helpful for insomnia, anxiety, migraine, and chronic pain. I have included TCH in previous sections, where applicable. Some examples include:

>> **Drugs:** Amitriptyline (Elavil, Vanatrip), doxepin (Silenor, Sinequan), nortriptyline (Aventyl, Pamelor), trimipramine (Surmontil)

>> **Herbs:** Black cohosh (*Actaea racemosa* or *Cimicifuga racemosa*), chamomile (*Matricaria recutita, Chamaemelum nobile*), chasteberry (*Vitex agnus-castus*), lavender (*Lavandula*), passionflower (*Passiflora incarnata*), saffron (*Crocus sativus*)

>> **TCH:** Guan Ye Lian Qiao (*Herba hypericum*), He Huan Pi (*Cortex albiziae*), Xiao Mai (*Fructus tritici*)

WARNING

Depending on their use, combining medicines in this category and with medicines from related categories (see depression, insomnia, and anxiety) can magnify side effects ranging from drowsiness to motor and cognitive impairment to anxiety.

Appendix A

Glossary

A1C: A blood test that measures an average of glucose levels over the past three months. Also known as *hemoglobin A1c (HbA1c)*.

Accreditation: Certification, of sorts, that an educational institution maintains standards in its course offerings that qualify graduates for admission to higher education or more specialized institutions for further study, or for professional practice.

Accreditation Commission for Acupuncture and Herbal Medicine (ACAHM): The U.S. national organization responsible for reviewing and evaluating Traditional Chinese Medicine (TCM) programs and institutions for accreditation.

Acupuncture: A TCM therapy where a practitioner stimulates specific points on the body, usually by inserting very fine needles into the skin and underlying tissues, to control pain and other symptoms.

Acupuncture and TCM Board of Reproductive Medicine (ABORM): A nonprofit organization that provides training, education, and certification in the use of Traditional Chinese Medicine in the field of Reproductive Health.

Acupuncture for Seniors Act: Legislation that, if passed by the U.S. Congress, would allow the Centers for Medicare & Medicaid Services to recognize acupuncturists as direct providers.

Acupuncturists Without Borders: Nonprofit organization that provides trauma-informed care, typically through auricular acupuncture, to communities impacted by natural disasters, human conflict, environmental devastation, poverty, and social injustice.

Adhesion: Abnormal scar tissue that can form after injury, infection, inflammation, or surgery, and binds tissues or organs that normally aren't physically connected.

Adrenaline: A hormone and neurotransmitter made by your body during times of excitement or stress, also known as *epinephrine*.

Allergic rhinitis: Inflammation and swelling inside the nose caused by seasonal allergies, also called *hay fever*.

Allopathic medicine: A system where medical doctors and other health-care professionals (such as nurses, pharmacists, and therapists) treat symptoms and diseases by using drugs, radiation, or surgery. Also called *biomedicine, conventional medicine, mainstream medicine, orthodox medicine,* and *Western medicine*.

American College of Traditional Chinese Medicine (ACTCM): Founded in 1980, ACTCM was one of the oldest and most respected TCM colleges in the U.S. It was the first to award a Master of Science in Traditional Chinese Medicine (MSTCM) in 1986 and achieved ACAHM accreditation in 1991. Acquired by the California Institute of Integral Studies (CIIS) in 2015, it established the first professional doctorate in acupuncture and Chinese medicine (DACM) that state and national accreditation authorities recognized. The college officially closed in 2024.

American Consortium for Integrative Medicine & Health: An international community of academic health centers and systems advocating and advancing the practice of whole health, with expertise in research, clinical care, and education on integrative medicine.

American Psychiatric Association (APA): The main professional organization of psychiatrists and trainee psychiatrists in the United States, with a focus on research, education, training, and advocacy.

American Society of Acupuncturists (ASA): A consortium of state acupuncture associations offering advocacy, awareness, networking, and professional development opportunities for TCM practitioners in the U.S.

American Society of Addiction Medicine (ASAM): A medical society of more than 8,000 physicians, clinicians, and related professionals who specialize in addiction medicine.

Analgesic: A type of medication used to relieve different types of pain by reducing inflammation or changing how the brain senses pain. Also called a *painkiller.*

Andropause: Occurs when testosterone production declines in men, sometimes causing uncomfortable physical and emotional symptoms. Also known as *male menopause.* See *Testosterone.*

Anorexia nervosa: An eating disorder characterized by an obsession with being thin — with a distorted body image, an extreme fear of obesity, and reduced food consumption — leading to a significantly low body weight.

Antiangiogenic: A substance used to prevent the formation and differentiation of blood vessels. In cancer treatment, it is used to slow or stop tumor growth.

Anticoagulant: A substance used to prevent and treat blood clots in blood vessels and the heart. Also called a *blood thinner.*

Anticoagulation: The process of reducing or preventing blood from clotting.

Antidiabetic: A substance used to address diabetes.

Antigen: Any substance that causes an immune response in the body against that substance, such as toxins, chemicals, bacteria, or viruses.

Antimetastatic: A substance that prevents the spread of a cancer from the initial site to another part of the body, such as keeping cancer cells from spreading from the breast to the lung.

Antioxidant: A substance that protects cells from daily damage caused by *free radicals* (unstable molecules formed during the normal processing of oxygen).

Antiplatelet: A substance that prevents or inhibits platelets from sticking to each other. See *platelet.*

Antiseizure: A substance that prevents or counteracts seizures.

Apoptosis: A molecular process inside a cell that leads to its death. One method that the body uses to get rid of unneeded or abnormal cells.

Aromatherapy: A type of complementary and alternative medicine that uses plant oils that have strong, pleasant scents (or aromas) to promote relaxation, a sense of well-being, and healing.

Asian bodywork therapy: Traditional Asian bodywork therapies, such as Japanese shiatsu, Thai bodywork, tui na, acupressure, and others, are used to relieve pain and improve well-being based on TCM principles.

Assisted reproduction technology (ART): A therapy that involves working with sperm and eggs or embryos in a laboratory (*in vitro*) with the goal of producing a pregnancy. See *In vitro fertilization.*

Attention-deficit hyperactivity disorder (ADHD): A disorder characterized by poor or short attention span and/or excessive activity and impulsiveness inappropriate for a person's age that interferes with their functioning or development.

Auriculotherapy: A type of acupuncture applied to specific points on the outer ear to control pain and other symptoms. Also known as *auricular acupuncture* or *ear acupuncture.*

Autonomic nervous system: The part of the nervous system that controls the muscles of the internal organs (such as the heart, blood vessels, lungs, stomach, and intestines) and glands (such as salivary glands and sweat glands). This system regulates certain body processes, such as blood pressure and the rate of breathing, and it works automatically (autonomously), without a person's conscious effort.

Autophagy: A process where a cell breaks down and destroys old, damaged, or abnormal proteins and other substances in its *cytoplasm* (the fluid inside a cell).

Benzodiazepine: A type of drug used to relieve anxiety and insomnia. Benzodiazepines are also used to relax muscles and prevent seizures. Also called *benzos.*

Biliary colic: Intermittent abdominal pain caused by the gallbladder or bile ducts.

Blood: In TCM, one of the vital substances that contributes to body function and sustenance. See *Vital Three.*

Bloodletting: A medical procedure originating in ancient times that involves the removal of blood from a person to manage diseases and health conditions.

Body Fluid: In TCM, one of the vital substances that contributes to body function. See *Vital Three.*

Breech presentation: The position of a fetus or baby where the feet or bottom are the first to appear at the exit of the womb.

Bulimia nervosa: An eating disorder characterized by eating large amounts of food (or *binge eating*), followed by attempts to make up for the overeating by vomiting, fasting, or exercising.

Cannabis: The dried leaves and flowering tops of the *Cannabis sativa* or *Cannabis indica* plant that contain active chemicals that affect various systems in the body, including the central nervous and immune systems. Also called *marijuana.*

Carboplatin: A drug used to treat advanced ovarian cancer in patients who have not been treated before or who have come back after treatment with other anticancer drugs.

Cardiovascular diseases: A group of blood and heart disorders that can lead to heart attack and stroke.

Cauterization: A medical technique that uses heat or chemicals to burn or destroy tissue.

Central nervous system (CNS): Network of nerves that send messaging between the brain and the spinal cord.

Cerebral cortex: The outer layer of the brain that functions mainly in coordinating sensory and motor information. Also called *gray matter.*

Chemotherapy: Treatment that uses drugs to stop the growth of cancer cells, either by killing the cells or by stopping them from dividing.

Chronic obstructive pulmonary disease (COPD): A type of lung disease marked by permanent damage to tissues in the lungs, making it hard to breathe.

CINV: Chemotherapy-induced nausea and vomiting. See *Chemotherapy.*

Circulatory system: The system that includes the heart and blood vessels and moves blood throughout the body.

Clean Needle Technique (CNT): An established protocol for safe and sanitary use and disposal of acupuncture needles; a practitioner needs CNT certification to receive a license and practice acupuncture in the U.S.

Codeine: An opioid drug that treats mild to moderate pain, cough, and diarrhea. See *Opioid.*

Cognitive impairment: Problems with a person's ability to think, learn, remember, use judgment, and make decisions.

Collaterals: In TCM, smaller supplemental channels to the meridians through which Qi flows in the body. See *Meridians.*

Comorbidity: The condition of having two or more unrelated diseases at the same time.

Complementary and alternative medicine (CAM): A term used to describe a non-standard medical product or practice used together with (*complementary*) or instead of (*alternative*) standard medical care.

Computed tomography (CT) scan: A procedure that uses a computer linked to an X-ray machine to take a series of detailed pictures of areas inside the body.

Confucianism: A system of thought and behavior developed by the Chinese philosopher and scholar Confucius (551–479 BCE) that focuses on personal ethics and morality.

Continuing education unit (CEU): A measure of someone's participation in continuing education experiences (courses, seminars, workshops, hands-on instruction, and so on), often used to track professional development and maintain licenses or certifications.

Contraindication: Anything that provides a reason *not* to prescribe a particular drug or apply a treatment or procedure to a patient because that prescription, treatment, or procedure may cause harm to that patient.

Cortical homunculus: A distorted-looking image of a person's body that reflects corresponding areas of the brain's motor and sensory cortexes.

Cortisol: An essential hormone made and released by the adrenal glands that affects almost every organ and tissue in the body; it regulates a variety of critical processes, such as how the body uses *glucose* (sugar) for energy, how your body responds to stress, and how the body sleeps and wakes.

Council of Colleges of Acupuncture and Herbal Medicine (CCAHM): U.S. national organization that sets curriculum and educational standards for TCM programs and institutions.

Cultural Revolution (China): A decade-long sociopolitical movement from 1966 to 1976, initiated by Mao Zedong to purge what he described as "capitalist and traditional elements" from Chinese society and reassert his authority.

Cupping: A TCM procedure in which you place a rounded glass or plastic cup upside down over an area of the body, creating suction that increases circulation.

Decoction: A concentrated extract of an herb or combination of herbs that you obtain by boiling the herb(s) in water.

Depression: A mental condition with symptoms of ongoing feelings of sadness, despair, loss of energy, and difficulty dealing with normal daily life.

Detoxification: The removal of a harmful substance (such as a poison or toxin); the process of weaning someone, such as a drug user or an alcoholic, off an addictive substance in the body or from dependence on or addiction to that substance.

Diabetes: A condition where the body can't use glucose normally, resulting in too much glucose in the blood, which can lead to serious illness.

Digestive system: The organs that take in food and liquids and break them down into substances that the body can use for energy, growth, and tissue repair.

Diuretic: A type of drug that causes the kidneys to make more urine.

Dopamine: A neurotransmitter made in brain cells (called *neurons*) that plays a role in the brain's reward system and affects many body functions, including memory, movement, motivation, mood, attention, and more. See *Neuron*.

Dry needling: A treatment that uses thin needles to address pain and movement issues associated with *myofascial* (muscles and their connective tissue) trigger points. See *fascia*.

Dysentery (bacterial): A disease marked by frequent and often painful passage of small amounts of stool that contain blood, pus, and mucus; caused by an infection of *shigella* bacteria. Also known as *shigellosis*.

Dysmenorrhea: Cramps or pain in the lowest part of the abdomen, a few days before, during, or after a menstrual period.

Ectopic pregnancy: A pregnancy in which a fertilized egg attaches in the wrong place, such as in a fallopian tube. See *Fallopian tubes*.

Electrostimulation: Use of electric current as therapy to stimulate healing in body tissue.

Embryology: A branch of biology dealing with embryos and their development.

Endocrine system: The glands and organs that make hormones, which serve as the body's chemical messengers and influence nearly every cell, organ, and function in the body.

Endometriosis: A noncancerous condition in which tissue that is like *endometrial* (membrane lining the uterus) tissue grows in abnormal places in the abdomen.

Endorphin: A type of neurotransmitter made in the body that can relieve pain and produce a feeling of well-being.

Enzyme: A protein that speeds up chemical reactions, such as digestion, blood clotting, and cell growth, in the body.

Essence: In TCM, one of the vital substances that contributes to body function. See *Vital Three*.

Estrogen: A type of hormone made by the body that helps develop and maintain female sex characteristics and the growth of long bones.

Evidence of coverage (EOC): A legal document that details the specific terms and conditions of an insurance policy, including what services the policy covers, how much the policyholder pays, and how the plan operates.

Fallopian tubes: Passageways for an egg and a sperm to meet and for a fertilized egg to make its way to the uterus.

Fascia: A sheet of connective tissue covering or binding together body structures (such as muscles).

Fentanyl: An opioid drug used to treat severe pain in people who have chronic conditions, such as cancer, who don't get relief from less potent opioids. Also used to treat pain after surgery. See *Opioid*.

Fibroids: A noncancerous tumor of the uterus that's composed of muscle and fibrous tissue.

Fibromyalgia: A condition characterized by poor sleep, fatigue, mental cloudiness, and widespread aching and stiffness in soft tissues, including muscles, tendons, and ligaments.

Five Elements Theory: Chinese philosophical theory organizing all natural phenomena into five main categories or patterns—Earth, Metal, Water, Wood, and Fire; used in TCM, martial arts, feng shui, and various systems of thought and behavior.

Flexible Spending Account (FSA): A U.S. employee benefit that allows an employee to set aside money from their paycheck (pre-tax) to pay for healthcare and dependent care expenses.

fMRI: Functional magnetic resonance imaging, which focuses on blood flow in the brain to measure brain activity. See *Magnetic resonance imaging.*

Follicle-stimulating hormone (FSH): A hormone produced by the pituitary gland that signals the ovaries and testes to make other hormones that lead to the sexual transformation of girls to women and boys to men during puberty. Works with luteinizing hormone (LH). Also related to pregnancy and menstruation. See *Luteinizing hormone.*

Gout: A condition marked by increased levels of uric acid in the blood, joints, and tissue that causes arthritis and inflammation.

Gua: A Chinese word meaning to scrape or scratch. See *Gua sha.*

Gua sha: A TCM technique in which a practitioner uses a smooth-edged tool to press and stroke on lubricated skin to improve blood circulation and relieve pain.

Hallucinogen: A class of drugs that cause serious distortions in people's perceptions and thinking, such as hallucinations.

Hamilton Rating Scale for Depression (HAM-D): Rating scale used to assess the severity of depression. See *Depression.*

Healthcare-associated infection (HAI): Infections that a person can get while in a healthcare facility. Also known as *nosocomial infections.*

Health Savings Account (HSA): A type of personal savings account used to pay certain health care costs.

Health Reimbursement Account (HRA): An employer-funded group health benefit that provides tax-free reimbursement for qualified medical expenses up to a fixed dollar amount per year. Also known as *Health Reimbursement Arrangement.*

Hemerology: A system of obtaining spiritual insight that evaluates specific time periods, such as seasons, months, days, or hours, to predict the fortunate or unfortunate outcome of events or actions taken during those times.

Hemodynamic: Relating to or functioning in the mechanics of blood circulation.

Herbology: The study of herbal medicine.

Heroin: A highly addictive opioid, made from morphine, that Western medicine practitioners used to treat severe pain at the turn of the 20th century; now illegal to use or sell in the U.S. See *Opioid.*

Hippocratic Corpus: A collection of ancient Greek medical papers.

Histamine: A type of neurotransmitter released by the immune system during allergic reactions.

Homeopathy: An alternative approach to medicine based on the belief that natural substances, prepared specially and used in very small amounts, restore health. Also called *homeopathic medicine.*

Homeostasis: A state of balance among all the body systems needed for the body to survive and function correctly.

Hydrocodone: An opioid drug used to treat moderate-to-severe pain, as well as cough. See *Opioid.*

Hypertension: A health condition in which the force of blood against the artery walls is too high; more commonly known as *high blood pressure.*

Hypotension: A health condition in which the force of blood against the artery walls is too low; more commonly known as *low blood pressure.*

***I Ching* (*Book of Changes*):** Ancient Chinese philosophical text fundamental to both Confucianism and Taoism. See *Confucianism* and *Taoism.*

Immune system: A network of cells, tissues, organs, and the substances that they make that helps the body fight infections and other diseases.

Immunotherapy: A type of therapy that uses substances to stimulate or suppress the immune system to help the body fight cancer, infection, and other diseases.

Inhalant: A substance (such as an allergen or medication) that you breathe in.

Integrative medicine: An approach to medical care that recognizes the benefit of combining conventional therapies (such as drugs and surgery) with safe and effective complementary therapies (such as acupuncture and yoga). See *Allopathic medicine* and *Complementary and alternative medicine.*

Integumentary system: The body's outer layer that consists of skin, hair, nails, and glands.

Intrauterine insemination (IUI): A reproductive technology that involves selecting the most active sperm, then placing them directly in the uterus through a tube inserted into the cervix.

In vitro fertilization (IVF): A reproductive technology that fertilizes eggs in a laboratory.

Irritable bowel syndrome: A disorder of the intestines that has symptoms such as abdominal pain, bloating, and changes in a person's bowel habits.

Letter of Medical Necessity (LMN): A formal document provided by a licensed healthcare provider that explains why a specific treatment, product, piece of medical equipment, medication, or medical service is essential for a patient's health and well-being.

Leukocyte: A type of blood cell made in the bone marrow and found in the blood and lymph tissue that functions as part of the body's immune system. Also known as *white blood cells* or *WBCs*.

Leukopenia: A condition where the number of leukocytes in the blood is lower than normal. See *Leukocyte*.

Liraglutide: A medication that treats Type-2 diabetes that can also help prevent a stroke or heart attack in people who have diabetes. See *Diabetes*.

Luteinizing hormone (LH): A hormone released by the pituitary gland that stimulates ovulation in women and the development of interstitial tissue in men's testes. Works with follicle-stimulating hormone (FSH) to trigger puberty. See *Follicle-stimulating hormone*.

Lyme disease: A bacterial infection transmitted by ticks in the U.S.

Lymphatic system: The tissues and organs that help the body fight infection and disease.

Lymphocyte: A type of leukocyte that makes antibodies, helps kill tumor cells, and controls immune responses. See *Leukocyte*.

Magnetic resonance imaging (MRI): A procedure that uses radio waves, a powerful magnet, and a computer to make a series of detailed pictures of areas inside the body.

Mastitis: A condition in which breast tissue is inflamed.

Materia medica: Substances used in making medical remedies; a branch of medical science that deals with the sources, nature, properties, and preparation of drugs.

Medical acupuncture: An adaptation of acupuncture administered by medical doctors and doctors of osteopathy.

Melanoma: A form of cancer that begins in *melanocytes* (cells that make melanin, which gives skin its color).

Meridians: One of 20 channels that form a network through which Qi flows, connecting the body's acupuncture sites. Also called *vessels*. See *Qi*.

Mind-body medicine: An approach to healing that acknowledges and uses thoughts, emotions, and spirituality to influence physical health.

Mitogen-activated protein kinases: A family of enzymes that play a crucial role in converting one type of cellular signal or energy into another.

Monkeypox: A disease similar to smallpox that is caused by a virus. Also known as *mpox*.

Morphine: An opioid drug used to treat moderate-to-severe pain. See *Opioid*.

Moxa: A TCM herb used for the TCM therapy of moxibustion; also known as Chinese mugwort (*Artemisia argyi*). See *Moxibustion*.

Moxibustion: A type of TCM heat therapy where the practitioner burns moxa on or above the skin to warm and stimulate an acupuncture point or affected area. See *Moxa*.

Musculoskeletal system: System that provides form, stability, and movement to the human body. It consists of bones (the skeleton), muscles, tendons, ligaments, joints, cartilage, and other connective tissue.

NADA protocol: A standard ear acupuncture protocol developed by the National Acupuncture Detoxification Association that's used in trauma, addiction, and mental health therapy. See *National Acupuncture Detoxification Association.*

National Acupuncture Detoxification Association (NADA): U.S. organization that trains people in the NADA protocol to treat trauma, substance abuse, and mental health conditions. See *NADA protocol.*

National Certification Commission for Acupuncture and Oriental Medicine (NCCAOM) [now National Certification Board of Acupuncture and Herbal Medicine (NCBAHM)]: U.S. organization responsible for testing and certifying practitioners in acupuncture, herbology, Asian bodywork therapy, and Oriental medicine.

National Council on Problem Gambling: U.S. nonprofit organization that provides education on and builds awareness of the economic and social costs associated with gambling addiction.

Naturopathy: A system of disease prevention and treatment that avoids drugs and surgery.

Neuro-acupuncture: A type of acupuncture applied to the head. Also known as *scalp acupuncture*. See *Acupuncture.*

Neurobiology: A branch of life sciences that deals with the anatomy, physiology, and pathology of the nervous system.

Neuron: A grayish or reddish granular cell that's the basic functional unit of nervous tissue, transmitting and receiving nerve impulses.

Neuropathy: A nerve problem that causes pain, numbness, tingling, swelling, or muscle weakness in different parts of the body.

Nicotine: An addictive, poisonous chemical found in tobacco.

Nociceptor: A neuron that signals or senses pain. See Neuron.

Nonsteroidal anti-inflammatory drugs (NSAIDs): Medications that people use to decrease inflammation, reduce fever, and relieve pain.

Numerology: The study of the mystical or supernatural significance of numbers.

Nutraceuticals: A term commonly used in reference to a product derived from a food source that provides additional health benefits apart from basic nutritional value.

Obesity: A common, chronic disease characterized by an abnormally high, unhealthy amount of body fat.

Obsessive-compulsive disorder (OCD): An anxiety disorder where a person has intrusive ideas, thoughts, or images that occur repeatedly, and where they feel they must perform certain behaviors over and over again.

Opioid: A class of pain-relieving drugs derived from the opium poppy that have a high potential for misuse and addiction.

Oriental medicine: Another name for Traditional Chinese Medicine (TCM).

Osteoarthritis: A chronic disorder that causes damage to cartilage and surrounding tissues; characterized by pain, stiffness, and loss of function in the body's joints, mainly in the hands, knees, hips, and spine.

Osteoporosis: A condition where the amount and thickness of bone tissue decreases.

Over-the-counter (OTC) drugs: Medications that you can purchase without a prescription.

Ovulation: The release of an egg from an ovary during the menstrual cycle.

Oxidative stress: A condition that occurs when the body doesn't have enough antioxidants to remove unstable molecules, called *free radicals,* whose presence in the body can lead to cell and tissue damage. See *Antioxidant.*

Oxycodone: An opioid drug used to relieve moderate to severe pain. See *Opioid.*

Paclitaxel: A chemotherapy drug used alone or with other drugs to treat specific cancers, such as advanced ovarian cancer, certain types of breast cancer, and non-small cell lung cancer.

Palpate: To examine by touch, especially medically.

Parasympathetic nervous system: The part of the nervous system that slows the heart, dilates blood vessels, decreases pupil size, increases digestive juices, and relaxes muscles in the gastrointestinal tract; it leads the body to *rest and relax* or *rest and digest.*

Parkinson's disease: A slowly progressive degenerative disorder of the brain and spinal cord characterized by difficulty controlling or inability to control movement.

Paroxetine: A selective serotonin reuptake inhibitor (SSRI) drug used to treat depression and anxiety disorders; brand name *Paxil.* See *Selective serotonin reuptake inhibitor.*

Pathogenesis: The origination and development of a disease.

Pathology: The study of diseases and how they affect the body, particularly by testing and examining tissues, organs, and fluids; the typical behavior or progression of a disease.

Periarthritis: A condition characterized by a buildup of calcium in the soft tissue around a joint, causing inflammation that leads to pain or stiffness (instead of within the cartilage or bone of the joint itself, as happens with arthritis).

Peripheral nervous system: A network of nerves throughout the body that carries messages to and from the central nervous system (the brain and spinal cord). See *Central nervous system*.

Phagocyte: A type of leukocyte that kills and eats invading organisms and removes dead cells. See *Leukocyte*.

Pharmacokinetics: The activity of drugs in the body over a period of time, including how the body absorbs, distributes, and excretes them.

Phobia: An extreme, irrational fear of something that may cause a person to panic.

Placebo: An inactive substance or treatment that looks the same and is administered in the same way as an active drug or treatment; used to test the efficacy and safety of the active drug or treatment.

Polycystic ovary syndrome (PCOS): A condition affecting females caused by an overproduction of *androgens* (male hormones), resulting in excess hair growth, irregular menstruation, infertility, and obesity, among other issues.

Polymodal receptors: Sensory nerve receptors that respond to a wide variety of stimuli, including mechanical, chemical, and thermal inputs.

Postpartum depression (PPD): A feeling of extreme sadness and loss of interest in usual activities experienced by the childbearer during the first year after delivery and lasting more than 2 weeks. See *Depression*.

Post-traumatic stress disorder (PTSD): An anxiety disorder that develops in reaction to physical injury or severe mental or emotional distress, such as military combat, violent assault, natural disaster, or other life-threatening events.

Prednisone: A steroid drug used to reduce inflammation and lower the body's immune response.

Preeclampsia: Hypertension that develops after the 20th week of pregnancy, or a worsening of existing hypertension during this time. See *Hypertension*.

Prefrontal cortex: The outer layer (called *gray matter*) of the front of the brain that processes and regulates complex cognitive, emotional, and behavioral functioning. Also known as *the personality center of the brain*.

Prevalence: The percentage of a population that's affected with a particular disease at a given time.

Qi: Vital energy or life force in TCM theory that keeps a person's spiritual, emotional, mental, and physical health in balance.

Qigong: A form of traditional Chinese mind/body exercise and meditation that uses slow and precise body movements with controlled breathing and mental focusing to improve balance, flexibility, muscle strength, and overall health.

Radical: In written Chinese language, a basic character (similar to a word) that acts as a component of a more complex character.

Radiopathy: The use of high-energy radiation from X-rays, gamma rays, neutrons, protons, and other sources to kill cancer cells and shrink tumors.

Reciprocity: In the case of professional credentials, recognition by countries, states, or institutions of the validity of licenses or privileges granted by one another.

Remission: A decrease in or disappearance of signs and symptoms of cancer. Can also refer to a decrease in or disappearance of signs and symptoms of other chronic diseases.

Renal colic: Severe pain between the ribs and hip on the affected side that comes and goes every few minutes, usually from a urinary tract obstruction.

Reproductive system: The tissues, glands, and organs involved in producing children.

Respiratory system: The organs involved in the exchange of gases (oxygen in and carbon dioxide out) to support life.

Rheumatoid arthritis: A form of arthritis caused by the immune system attacking the body's tissues, in which joints, usually on the hands and feet, are inflamed, resulting in swelling, pain, and often joint damage or destruction.

Sciatica: Pain along the sciatic nerves that run from the lower back, through the buttocks, and down the legs, ending just below the knee. Also known as *lumbosacral radiculopathy*.

Scoliosis: A condition marked by a side-to-side curve of the backbone. The curve is usually shaped like an S or a C.

Sedative: A drug or substance used to calm a person down, relieve anxiety, or help a person sleep.

Selective serotonin reuptake inhibitors (SSRIs): A type of drug used to treat depression, anxiety, and some forms of pain.

Serotonin: A chemical that's both a *neurotransmitter* (sending messages between nerves and the brain) and a hormone; it affects various body functions, such as mood, sleep, digestion, nausea, wound healing, bone health, blood clotting, and sexual desire.

Sha: A skin rash that appears as petechiae or tiny red spots that result from a gua sha treatment. See *Gua sha*.

Silymarin: A substance obtained from milk thistle seeds that's being studied in the prevention of liver damage caused by certain cancer treatments.

Spinal stenosis: Narrowing of the spinal canal.

Society for Acupuncture Research: International organization that evaluates and improves research for acupuncture and other TCM therapies.

Steroid: A prescription medication that reduces inflammation. Also called *corticosteroids* or *glucocorticoids*.

Substance Abuse and Mental Health Services Administration (SAMHSA): Agency within the U.S. Department of Health and Human Services that leads public health efforts to advance the behavioral and mental health of the nation.

Sympathetic nervous system: The part of the nervous system that activates your fight or flight response when you're stressed or in danger. This response includes increasing your heart rate, enlarging your pupils, and expanding your breathing capacity.

Sympathomimetic: A substance that mimics the physical effects of the sympathetic nervous system (the fight or flight response).

Systematic review: A rigorous and critical review and summary of research on a specific topic.

Tai chi: A form of traditional Chinese mind/body exercise and meditation that uses slow sets of body movements and controlled breathing; can improve balance, flexibility, muscle strength, and overall health.

Taoism: An ancient Chinese philosophy and religion founded by Lao Tzu in the 6th century BCE that instructs believers on how to exist in harmony with the universe. Also known as *Daoism*.

Teding Diancibo Pu (TDP): Therapeutic heat lamps used in TCM for pain relief and other health benefits. Teding Diancibo Pu translates to *special electromagnetic spectrum.* These lamps use a ceramic disc coated with 33 special minerals to regulate infrared radiation.

Tennis elbow: Inflammation of the elbow tendons and muscles that extend the hand backward and away from the palm.

Testicular microcirculation: The tiny network of blood vessels within the testicles that is crucial for delivering oxygen, nutrients, and hormones while also removing waste products.

Testosterone: A hormone made mainly in the *testes* (part of the male reproductive system) needed to develop and maintain male sex characteristics, such as facial hair, deep voice, and muscle growth. In women, testosterone is produced mostly in the ovaries and adrenal glands.

Thermoreceptors: A sensory neuron that detects and responds to changes in temperature.

Tincture: A medicinal substance mixed with or dissolved in alcohol.

Tonify: TCM term that means to invigorate, restore, refresh, or stimulate.

Traditional Chinese Herbs (TCH): The *materia medica* of TCM; Chinese herbs used for medicinal purposes.

Traditional Chinese Medicine (TCM): A medical system that originated in China around the 3rd century BCE; used for thousands of years to prevent, diagnose, and treat disease. Also called *Oriental medicine* or more recently, *Traditional East Asian Medicine* (TEAM).

Transcutaneous electrical nerve stimulation (TENS): A procedure in which a device applies mild electric currents to some areas of the skin by using adhesive pads.

Tricyclic antidepressants (TCAs): A class of drugs used to treat symptoms of major depressive disorder.

Tubal factor: A type of female infertility caused by damage, blockage, or abnormalities in the fallopian tubes, which prevents the sperm from reaching the egg or the fertilized egg from implanting in the uterus. See *Fallopian tube.*

Tui na: Chinese massage that uses kneading, pressing, rolling, shaking, and stretching of the body.

Urinary system: The organs that make urine and remove it from the body.

Vessels: See *Meridians.*

Visual Analog Scale (VAS): A scale that uses images, words, and/or numbers to measure the severity or intensity of pain.

Vital Three: Qi, Blood, and Body Fluid; the three vital or fundamental substances that maintain the activities and functions of the body in TCM theory.

Yang: The active force in nature that complements and counterbalances Yin to make up all aspects of life according to Taoist theory. See *Yin.*

Yin: The passive force in nature that complements and counterbalances Yang to make up all aspects of life according to Taoist theory. See *Yang.*

Appendix B

Resources

Whether you want to explore more about Traditional Chinese Medicine (TCM), find a practitioner, or learn more about the conditions in this book, this appendix includes links to organizations, associations, and sources of information that I've come to trust.

TIP

Because you can find so much information out there, I recommend finding one or two sources that you trust to support your healthcare and self-care choices. I've listed my go-to sites that I don't mention elsewhere in the book at the end of this appendix.

I organized the resources in the following sections by chapter so that you can have a context for the information.

Chapter 1: Looking at Health through a TCM Lens

>> Cleveland Clinic — Health Library: https//my.clevelandclinic.org/health

>> National Institutes of Health: https://www.nih.gov/

>> Mawangdui Exhibit: https://www.hnmuseum.com/en/content/changsha-mawangdui-han-dynasty-tombs-exhibition

>> Andrew Weil Center for Integrative Medicine: https://awcim.arizona.edu/

>> World Health Organization: https://www.who.int/

Chapter 3: Accessing TCM Professionals

>> National Certification Commission for Acupuncture and Oriental Medicine [now National Certification Board for Acupuncture and Herbal Medicine]: https://www.ncbahm.org/

>> California Acupuncture Board: www.acupuncture.ca.gov

>> Council of Colleges of Acupuncture and Herbal Medicine: www.ccahm.org/ccaom

>> Accreditation Commission for Acupuncture and Herbal Medicine: www.acahm.org

>> American Society of Acupuncturists: www.asacu.org

>> Society for Acupuncture Research: www.acupunctureresearch.org

>> American Academy of Medical Acupuncture: www.medicalacupuncture.org

>> American Physical Therapy Association: https://www.apta.org

>> Board of Certification for the Athletic Trainer: https://bocatc.org

>> World Health Organization: https://www.who.int

>> People's Organization of Community Acupuncture: www.pocacoop.com

>> Veterans Health Administration — Whole Health: www.va.gov/wholehealth

Chapter 4: Understanding Acupuncture

>> Acupuncture Now Foundation: www.acunow.org

>> U.S. Food and Drug Administration: www.fda.gov

>> World Health Organization: https://www.who.int

>> American Academy of Medical Acupuncture: www.medicalacupuncture.org

Chapter 5: Examining Other TCM Therapies

» National Certification Commission for Acupuncture and Oriental Medicine [now National Certification Board for Acupuncture and Herbal Medicine]: https://www.ncbahm.org

» Cochrane Database of Systematic Reviews: https://www.cochranelibrary.com

» Andrew Weil Center for Integrative Medicine: https://awcim.arizona.edu

Chapter 6: Knowing What to Expect from TCM Treatment

» National Certification Commission for Acupuncture and Oriental Medicine [now National Certification Board for Acupuncture and Herbal Medicine]: https://www.ncbahm.org

» Council of Colleges of Acupuncture and Herbal Medicine: www.ccahm.org/ccaom

Chapter 7: Relieving Pain

» World Health Organization: https://www.who.int

» National Health Interview Survey: www.cdc.gov/nchs/nhis/index.html

» Pain Management Best Practices Inter-Agency Task Force Report: www.hhs.gov/opioids/prevention/pain-management-options/index.html

» U.S. Centers for Disease Control and Prevention: www.cdc.gov

» American College of Physicians: www.acponline.org

» Centers for Medicare and Medicaid Services: www.cms.gov

Chapter 8: Managing Addictions and Mental Health

>> U.S. Centers for Disease Control and Prevention: www.cdc.gov

>> American Society of Addiction Medicine: www.asam.org

>> Substance Abuse and Mental Health Services Administration [National Survey on Drug Use and Health]: www.samhsa.gov

>> National Council of Problem Gambling: www.ncpgambling.org

>> National Acupuncture Detoxification Association: www.acudetox.com

>> American Lung Association: www.lung.org

>> National Youth Tobacco Survey: www.fda.gov/tobacco-products/youth-and-tobacco/results-annual-national-youth-tobacco-survey

>> American Psychological Association: www.apa.org

>> American Psychiatric Association: www.psychiatry.org

>> Acupuncturists Without Borders: www.acuwithoutborders.org

Chapter 9: Supporting Reproduction

>> Cleveland Clinic — Health Library: http://my.clevelandclinic.org/health

>> The American Society for Reproductive Medicine [76th Scientific Congress of the American Society for Reproductive Medicine]: https://www.asrm.org

>> World Health Organization: www.who.int

>> The Acupuncture and TCM Board of Reproductive Medicine: www.aborm.org

Chapter 10: Supplementing Cancer Treatment

>> American Cancer Society: www.cancer.org

>> Memorial Sloan Kettering Cancer Center: www.mskcc.org

- » National Comprehensive Cancer Network: www.nccn.org
- » National Cancer Institute: www.cancer.gov

Chapter 11: Ten Ways to Eat the TCM Way

- » National Resources Defense Council: www.nrdc.org

Chapter 13: Ten (or So) Products Your Medicine Cabinet

- » U.S. Food and Drug Administration: www.fda.gov
- » National Institutes of Health, Office of Dietary Supplements: https://ods.od.nih.gov
- » Better Business Bureau: https://www.bbb.org
- » World Health Organization [Good Manufacturing Practices]: https://www.who.int
- » American Herbal Products Association: www.ahpa.org
- » Consumer Healthcare Products Association: www.chpa.org
- » Council for Responsible Nutrition: www.crnusa.org
- » United Natural Products Alliance: www.unpa.com
- » Consumer Reports: www.consumerreports.org
- » Environmental Working Group: www.ewg.org

My Go-To Information Sources

- » About Herbs, Botanicals & Other Products, Memorial Sloan Kettering Cancer Center: www.mskcc.org

- >> American College of Obstetricians and Gynecologists Women's Health Guide: www.acog.org/womens-health

- >> Andrew Weil Center for Integrative Medicine: http://awcim.arizona.edu

- >> Blue Zones: www.bluezones.com

- >> Herbal Academy: www.theherbalacademy.com

- >> Mayo Clinic: www.mayoclinic.org

- >> Merck Manual: www.merckmanuals.com

- >> National Center for Complementary and Integrative Health: www.nccih.nih.gov

- >> National Center for Complementary and Integrative Health — Herbs at a Glance: www.nccih.nih.gov/health/herbsataglance

- >> Office of Dietary Supplements, National Institutes of Health: http://ods.od.nih.gov

- >> Office of Research on Women's Health, National Institutes of Health: http://orwh.od.nih.gov

- >> Wellness Toolkits, National Institutes of Health: www.nih.gov/health-information/your-healthiest-self-wellness-toolkits

Index

bones, 41

botanicals, 248. *See also* herbs

bowel movements, medicinals for, 243

brain, 41, 78, 87, 143, 172

breast cancer, 208

breastfeeding, 188

breathwork, 117

  Qigong, 17, 117–120, 173, 174, 176, 207, 225

  tai chi, 117, 119–120, 176, 207, 225

breech presentation, 188

C

caffeine, 254

CALE. *See* California Acupuncture Licensing Exam

California Acupuncture Licensing Exam (CALE), 57

CAM. *See* complementary and alternative medicine

cancer development, 195

cancer-related fatigue (CRF), 205–207

cancer treatment, 191–192. *See also* ovarian cancer (case study)

  diagnosis, 195–196

  post-treatment care, 210

  resources, 280–281

  side effects, easing, 205–210

Cang Er Zi San (Wan), 245

Cang Zhu (Rhizoma Atractylodis), 256

cannabidiol (Epidiolex), 257

cannabis (*Cannabis sativa*), 257

carbamazepine (Epitol, Tegretol), 257

carboplatin, 195

CCAHM. *See* Council of Colleges of Acupuncture and Herbal Medicine

CDC. *See* Centers for Disease Control and Prevention

CE. *See* continuing education

Centers for Disease Control and Prevention (CDC), 141, 165

Centers for Medicare and Medicaid Services (CMS), 61, 141, 152–153

centralized pain, 143

central nervous system, 143

cerebral cortex, 87–88, 174

Ceylon cinnamon (*Cinnamomum zeylanicum*), 256

chamomile (*Matricaria recutita, Chamaemelum nobile*), 254, 257–260

channel(s), 72, 157

  functions of, 42–43

  mapping, 43–45

  points, 46–47

  properties of herbs, 103

character of pulse, 130

chasteberry (*Vitex agnus-castus*), 257, 260

chemotherapy, 195, 205

chemotherapy-induced nausea and vomiting (CINV), 209–210

Chen, Chao, 90

Cheng Zhong-Ling, 103

Che Qian Zi (*Semen plantaginis*), 256

Cheung, S.Y.C., 168

Chi. *See* Qi

Chinese Acupuncture and Moxibustion (CAM), 86, 96, 162, 171

Chinese Herbal Medicine: Materia Medica, 3rd Edition (Bensky et al.), 100, 103

Chinese herbology, 54

Chinese Materia Medica (*Zhong Hua Ben Cao*), 100

Chinese mugwort (*Artemisia argyi*), 96, 97

Chinese scalp acupuncture. *See* scalp acupuncture

Chirali, Ilkay Zihni, 110–111

CHPA. *See* Consumer Healthcare Products Association

chronic pain, 142, 143, 145

chronic tension headaches, 157

Chu, Judy, 61

Chuan Xiong Cha Tiao Wan, 244

Chuan Xiong (Rhizoma ligustici chuanxiong), 254

Chuan Xiong Wan. *See* Chuan Xiong Cha Tiao Wan

CIH. *See* complementary and integrative health

cilantro (*Coriandrum sativum*), 257

cilostazol (Pletal), 255

CINV. *See* chemotherapy-induced nausea and vomiting

citalopram (Celexa), 257

Citkovitz, Claudia, 187

Classical Chinese Medicine, 15, 88–89

Clean Needle Technique (CNT) certification, 59, 133–135

Clean Needle Technique Manual, The, 133–134

clinical trials, 14

clonazepam (Klonopin), 258, 259

clopidogrel (Plavix), 255

clothing for TCM treatment, 137–138

CMS. *See* Centers for Medicare and Medicaid Services

CNT. *See* Clean Needle Technique certification

coat on tongue, 128–129

cocaine, 254

Cochrane reviews, 116, 117

cold (*Han*)

  as environmental pathogen, 198

  and hot (balance), 34, 125, 192, 203, 209, 218–219

collaterals, 42, 45

community acupuncture clinics, 64, 133

complementary and alternative medicine (CAM), 10, 189

complementary and integrative health (CIH), 63, 65

Conception Vessel-6 (REN-6) point, 234–235

Confucianism, 90

Consumer Healthcare Products Association (CHPA), 249

Consumer Reports, 249

continuing education (CE), 53

cooking, food, 218–219

cordyceps fruiting body (*dong chong xia cao*), 206

corporeal soul, 163

cortical homunculus, 87–88

cortisol, 115, 173, 176

Corydalis Rhizoma (*yan hu suo*), 155, 158–159

cough, medicinals for, 246

Council for Responsible Nutrition (CRN), 249

Council of Colleges of Acupuncture and Herbal Medicine (CCAHM), 58–59, 133

counteracting relationship (Five Elements cycle), 29–30

counteraction theory, 109–110

CRF. *See* cancer-related fatigue

CRN. *See* Council for Responsible Nutrition

cupping, 17, 109–111, 131

  for back pain, 154–155

  for headaches, 160

  origins of, 109–110

  treatments, 110–111

cytotoxic T cells, 80

D

Da Huang, 243

Dampness (*Shi*), 197, 204

dandelion (*Taraxacum officinale*), 256

Dang Gui (Radix angelicae sinensis), 254, 255

Dan Shen (Radix salvia miltiorrhizae), 254, 258

Da Suan (Bulbus alli sativi), 255

DCFSA. *See* Dependent Care Flexible Spending Account

De acupunctura (Rhijne), 73

decoctions, 105–107

deficiency and excess (balance), 34–35, 203–204

delivery (childbirth), 187–188

Dependent Care Flexible Spending Account (DCFSA), 67

depression, 175–176

  antidepressants, 257–259

  herbs for relieving, 257–258

  postpartum, 188–189

De Shou Tian, 116

designated female at birth (DFAB), 180–183

designated male at birth (DMAB), 178–179

detoxification programs, 168–169

Deutsche Zeitschrift für Akupunktur (*German Journal of Acupuncture, The*), 85

DFAB. *See* designated female at birth

diagnosis, 122–130, 195–196

  appearance of tongue, 127–129

  emotional factors, 200–201

  environmental pathogens, 195–200

  feeling of pulse, 127, 129–130

  health history, 123

  ovarian cancer (case study), 203–204

  palpating, 127

  physical appearance, 127

  ten questions of, 124–127

diazepam (Valium), 258, 259

Dietary Supplement Health and Education Act (DSHEA) of 1994, 248

dietary supplements, 247

dieticians, 108

digestion, 230, 241–242

Diplomate of Acupuncture (Dipl. Ac.), 53

Diplomate of Asian Bodywork Therapy (Dipl. ABT), 54

Diplomate of Chinese Herbology (Dipl. C.H.), 54

Diplomate of Oriental Medicine (Dipl. O.M.), 54

dipyridamole (Persantine), 255

directional flow

  of food, 219

  of herbs, 103

Discussion of Cold Damage (*Shang Han Lun*), 100

distal points, acupuncture, 149

diuretics, 255–256

Divine Husbandman's Classic of the Materia Medica (*Shen Nong Ben Cao Jing*), 100

dizziness, 125

DMAB. *See* designated male at birth

dopamine (Intropin), 173, 254

dose-dense chemotherapy, 195

doxepin (Silenor, Sinequan), 260

drinking, 126

  liquids, with meals, 220–221

  Yin-Yang water, 221–222

Dr. Shir's Liniment, 247

drug overdose deaths, 165

drugs

for activation of nervous system, 254

anticoagulants, 254–255

antidepressants, 257–259

antiplatelets, 255

antiseizure medications, 257

anxiolytics, 258–259

for controlling blood sugar, 256

for insomnia, 258

interactions, 252–253

for lowering blood pressure, 255–256

off-label use, 259–260

dry needling, 91–92

Dryness (*Zao*), 197–198

DSHEA. *See* Dietary Supplement Health and Education Act of 1994

Du channel, 45

E

EAM. *See* East Asian Medicine

ear acupuncture, 84–86, 149, 158, 168–170

ear cauterization, 85

ear maps, 85, 86

ear seeds, 186, 237

Earth, 25–26, 196

and appetite, 208

spleen and stomach, 37

East Asian Medicine (EAM), 59

eating, 126. *See also* food

drinking liquids with meals, 220–221

resources, 281

seasonal, 217

sequential, 220

slow, 216

egg count/quality, 181

Egypt, spiritual guidance in, 13

Eight Balances, 31–35, 103, 122, 195. *See also* Five Elements; Vital Three

electrical stimulation (e-stim), 17, 158

electroacupuncture, 168, 173

Ellis, John, 116

embryology, 77

emotional disorders, 233

emotions, 126, 145, 200–201

empagliflozin (Jardiance), 256

Encyclopedia of Traditional Chinese Medicinal Substances (*Zhong Yao Da Ci Dian*), 100

endocrine system, 179

endometriosis, 183

endorphins, 184

energy, 126

boosting, 205

classification of food, 219

Conception Vessel-6 point, 234–235

environmental pathogens, 196–200

and back pain, 153–154

and osteoarthritis, 148–149

Environmental Working Group, 249

EOC. *See* evidence of coverage document

epinephrine (Adrenalin), 254

episodic tension headaches, 157

escitalopram (Lexapro), 257, 259

e-stim. *See* electrical stimulation

estrogen, 182

eszopiclone, 258

ethosuximide (Zarontin), 257

Evidence Map of Acupuncture, VHA, 84

evidence of coverage (EOC) document, 66

excess and deficiency (balance), 34–35, 203–204

EX-HN-3. *See* Extra Head and Neck-3 point

exterior and interior (balance), 35, 204

freshwater fish, 224

frozen food, 218

fruits, 217, 225

FSAs. *See* Flexible Spending Accounts

FSH. *See* follicle-stimulating hormone

Fu Ling (*Poria*), 256

functional food, 248

Fu organs, 36, 37, 40–41

furosemide (Lasix), 255

G

gabapentin (Horizant, Gralise, Neurontin), 257

gallbladder, 39

Gallbladder-14 (GB-14) point, 234

gallbladder channel, 45

gambling disorder, 166

Gan Jiang (Rhizoma zingiberis), 255

garlic (*Allium sativum*), 255, 256

GB-14. *See* Gallbladder-14 point

German chamomile (*Matricaria recutita*), 258, 259

Germany, TCM practices in, 16

ginger (*Zingiber officinale*), 208, 255, 256

ginseng (*Panax ginseng*), 256

glimepiride (Amaryl), 256

GMP. *See* Good Manufacturing Practices certification

Good Manufacturing Practices (GMP) certification, 249

Gou Teng (Ramulus uncariae cum uncis), 257

Greenwood, Michael, 85

Guan Ye Lian Qiao (*Herba hypericum*), 257, 260

gua sha, 17, 111–114, 131

DIY vs medical therapy, 113–114

origins of, 111–112

treatments, 112–113

Gui Ban (Plastrum testudinis), 259

guide tube insertion (acupuncture), 91

H

Hall of Impression. *See Yintang* point

head

Large Intestine-4 point, 228–229

neuro-acupuncture, 86–88, 158, 225

headaches, 125, 156–160

acupressure for, 234

identification of problem causing, 157–158

medicinals for, 243–244

primary, 156, 157

secondary, 156

signs of, 156

treatment of, 158–160

health history, 123

Health Reimbursement Arrangements (HRAs), 67

Health Savings Accounts (HSAs), 67

heart, 39–40, 162–163, 171, 200

Heart channel, 44

heat (*Re*)

and cold (balance), 34, 125, 192, 203, 209, 218–219

as environmental pathogen, 200, 204

heat sensations, 208–209

He Huan Pi (Cortex albiziae), 257, 258, 260

helper T cells, 80

heparin, 254

herbal medicines, 248

herbs, 17, 100–107. *See also* Traditional Chinese Herbs (TCH)

  for activation of nervous system, 254

  for averting blood clots, 255

  for controlling blood sugar, 256

  drug–herb interactions, 253

  for insomnia, 258

  for lowering blood pressure, 255–256

  for relieving depression, 257–258

  for slowing blood clot formation, 254–255

  for stopping seizures, 257

  for treating anxiety, 259

heroin addiction, 168–169

HFNS. *See* hot flushes and night sweats

Hippocrates, 10, 101, 111

Hippocratic Corpus, 109

holistic medicine, 9–10

homeostasis, 172

Hong Hua (Flos carthami), 254

hormones

  activation of, 182–184

  hormonal disorders, 181

hospital systems, acupuncturists in, 65

hot flushes and night sweats (HFNS), 208–209

Hou Po (Cortex magnoliae officinalis), 255

HRAs. *See* Health Reimbursement Arrangements

HSAs. *See* Health Savings Accounts

Huangdi, Emperor, 73–74

Huang Di Nei Jing (Yellow Emperor's Inner Canon, The), 73–74, 88, 90, 96–97, 102, 108, 149, 171, 192, 235

Huang Lian (Rhizoma coptidis), 255

Huang Qi (Radix astragali), 256

hun, 163

hydrochlorothiazide (Esidrix), 255

I

ibuprofen, 243

ICD. *See* International Classification of Diseases

I Ching (Book of Changes), 90

IM. *See* integrative medicine

immune system, 144, 179

  activation, and acupuncture, 80–81

  definition of, 77

  mast cells, 152

  medicinals for boosting immunity, 245

incompatibility (drug interaction), 253

India, spiritual guidance in, 13

infections, prevention of, 134

inflammatory pain, 144, 145

informed consent, 135–136

infrared lamp therapy, 17

injection therapy, 91

Inner Gate/Pass point, 233–234

insomnia, 216–217

  acupressure for, 233

  drugs/herbs for treating, 258

insufficient Qi, 48, 157

insurance coverage for acupuncture, 66–68

integrative medicine (IM), 10

interacting relationship (Five Elements cycle), 28–29

interior and exterior (balance), 35, 204

Internal Wind, 199

International Classification of Diseases (ICD), 141

interneurons, 79

intrauterine insemination, 185

in vitro fertilization (IVF), 185–187

isoproterenol (Isuprel), 254

IVF. *See* in vitro fertilization

IVF cycle, 185–186

martial Qigong, 118

massage, 17, 115–116, 150, 159

mast cells, 152

Master Tung's Acupuncture, 89–90

mastitis, 188

materia medica, 11, 54, 100

Materia Medica of Medicinal Properties
    (*Yao xing ben cao*), 101

Mawangdui scrolls, 11–12, 117

medical Qigong, 118

Medical Revelations (*Yi Xue Xin Wu*), 103

Medicare, 61, 66

medicinals, TCM, 239–240.
    See also Traditional Chinese
    Herbs (TCH)

  for aches and pains, 246–247

  for boosting immunity, 245

  for bowel movements, 243

  children's version, 240

  choosing, 240–241, 247–248

  for cold/flu, 241

  for cough, 246

  for digestion, 241–242

  for headaches, 243–244

  modifications, 240

  resources, 281

  for runny nose, 244–245

  for sleep, 247

  for stopping bleeding, 246

Meditations (Marcus Aurelius), 73

menstrual disorders, 183

menstruation, 182

mental health, 161–162

  defining the Spirit, 162–163

  definition of, 166

  resources, 280

  treating the Spirit and sub-spirits, 164

mental health conditions, 164.
    See also addiction

  anxiety, 175–176, 258–259

  depression, 175–176, 257–259

  identification of, 166–167

  postpartum depression, 188–189

  seeking treatment for, 167

mental pain, 145

meridians. *See* channels

Mesopotamia, spiritual guidance in, 13

Metal, 25–26, 38, 196

metformin (Glucophage), 256

Middle of the Crook (*Weizhong*),
    232–233

migraine headaches, 157, 244

mind, 171

mind-body medicine, 14, 117

mineral salt (*Natrii Sulfas; mang xiao*), 104

miscarriage, 183–184

motor neurons, 79

movement, 115–117

  for cancer-related fatigue, 207

  Qigong, 17, 117–120, 173, 174,
    176, 207, 225

  tai chi, 117, 119–120, 176, 207, 225

moxa, 97–99, 186, 230

moxibustion, 11, 16, 54, 74, 75, 96–99.
    See also acupuncture

  for arthritis, 151

  for cancer-related fatigue, 206

  Chinese mugwort (*Artemisia argyi*), 96, 97

  methods, 98–99

  for reducing breech presentation, 188

  using with IVF, 186

mugwort (*Artemisia vulgaris*), 16

mutual accentuation (TCH combination),
    104

mutual counteraction (TCH combination), 104–105

mutual enhancement (TCH combination), 104

N

osteoarthritis, 146
  acupuncture for, 149–150
  and environmental pathogens, 148–149
  identification of, 147–149
  Qi stagnation, 148
  signs of, 146–147
ovarian cancer (case study), 193
  cancer-related fatigue, 205–207
  diagnosis, 195–196, 203–204
  easing nausea and vomiting, 209–210
  easing treatment side effects, 205–210
  increasing appetite, 208
  observed signs of, 202
  progression of, 193
  reducing post-treatment pain and
    neuropathy, 207–208
  symptoms of, 201–202
  turning down heat sensations, 208–209
  Western medicine approach, 195
ovarian factor, 180, 181
ovarian reserve, 181–183
overacting relationship (Five Elements
    cycle), 30–31
Oxenhandler, Harry, 76

P

paclitaxel, 104, 195
pain, 92, 117, 125, 141–142. *See also*
    acupressure
  acute, 142
  back, 152–156
  chronic, 142, 143, 145
  cost of, 145–146
  and discomfort, difference between, 142
  medicinals for, 246–247
  mental, 145
  osteoarthritis and joint pain, 146–152
  pregnancy, 184
  resources related to, 279
  sensing, 143–145
  during TCM treatments, 130–132
  types of, 142–143
  Visual Analog Scale, 159
Pain Management Best Practices
    Inter-Agency Task Force, 145–146
palpating, 127
papaya, 242–243
parasympathetic nervous system, 176
paroxetine (Paxil, Pexeva), 189, 257, 259
parsley (*Petroselinum crispum*), 256
passionflower (*Passiflora incarnata*), 257,
    259, 260
passive immunity, 80
patent medicines, 239
pathogenesis, 122, 123
pathological pain, 144
Paulus, Wolfgang, 186
PC-6. *See* Pericardium-6 point
PCOS. *See* polycystic ovary syndrome
Pei (Bi) Min Kan Wan, 245
People's Organization of Community
    Acupuncture (POCA), 64
pericardium (xin bao luo), 40
Pericardium-6 (PC-6) point, 233–234
Pericardium channel, 44
peripheral pain, 142
person-centered approach (Hippocrates),
    10
phagocytes, 80–81
pharmacokinetics, 252, 253
phenobarbital (Solfoton, Luminal), 257
phenytoin (Dilantin, Phenytek), 257

Small Intestine-3 (SI-3) point, 231–232

Small intestine channel, 44

Smart Seafood and Sustainable Fish Buying Guide, 224

Smith, Michael O., 169

smoking, 171

Society for Acupuncture Research (SAR), 61

soul, 163

Spain, TCM practices in, 16

spinal cord, 78

spine
  Small Intestine-3 point, 231–232
  spinal arthritis, 153–154

Spirit (*Shen*), 162, 164, 200

spiritual guidance, 13

spiritual Qigong, 118

spleen, 37, 163, 197

Spleen channel, 44

SSRIs. *See* selective serotonin reuptake inhibitors

ST-36. *See* Stomach-36 point

standard formulas, TCH, 107

state licensing boards, 57–58

Steinberg, Arthur, 75

stillbirth, 183–184

St. John's wort (*Hypericum perforatum*), 257, 258

stomach, 37

Stomach-36 (ST-36) point, 230–231

Stomach channel, 44

stool, 125

stress, 172
  reduction, therapies for, 173–174
  response, 172–173

Suan Zao Ren (Semin zizyphi spinosae), 258

sub-spirits, 162–164

Substance Abuse and Mental Health Services Administration (SAMHSA), 166, 167

substance use disorders (SUDs), 165, 166
  cost of, 167–168
  NADA protocol, 169–170, 225
  smoking, 171

SUDs. *See* substance use disorders

suicide, 165

Sun Si Miao, 108

sweating, 125

Swimming Dragon Qigong (*Taiyi You Long Gong*), 118

sympathetic nervous system, 254

sympathomimetic drugs, 254

synergism (drug interaction), 253

T

tai chi, 17, 117, 119–120, 225
  for anxiety/depression, 176
  for cancer-related fatigue, 207

Taiji, 32

tamoxifen, 208

Tan Balance Method, 90

Tan, Richard Teh-Fu, 90

Taoism, 22, 31–32, 90, 118

Tao Ren (Semen persicae), 254

taste properties of herbs, 102

Taxus brevifolia, 104

TCAs. *See* tricyclic antidepressants

T cells, 80

TCH. *See* Traditional Chinese Herbs

TCM. *See* Traditional Chinese Medicine

TDP. *See* Teding Diancibo Pu lamp therapy

Teding Diancibo Pu (TDP) lamp therapy, 17

temazepam, 258

temperature
  and food, 219
  properties, of herbs, 102
ten questions of diagnosis, 124–127
TENS. *See* transcutaneous electrical nerve stimulation
tension headaches, 156–157, 159
testicular microcirculation, 179
testosterone, 179, 182
Testudinis Plastrum (*gui ban*), 209
therapeutic action of herbs, 102–103
therapeutic principle of herbs, 103
Tian Ma (Rhizoma gastrodiae), 257
tinctures, 106–107
tirofiban (Aggrastat), 255
Tkach, Walter R., 75
tongue, appearance of, 127–129
topicals, 247
Traditional Chinese Herbs (TCH), 100–1007, 251–252
  for activation of nervous system, 254
  for arthritis, 151
  for averting blood clots, 255
  for back pain, 155–156
  for cancer-related fatigue, 206
  for cancer treatment pain, 207
  for chemotherapy-induced nausea and vomiting, 210
  for conditions related to female infertility, 183
  for controlling blood sugar, 256
  for female infertility, 182–183
  food as medicine, 101
  formulas, 104–107
  for headaches, 158–159
  for HFNS, 209
  for insomnia, 258
  for lowering blood pressure, 255–256
  for male infertility, 179
  practitioner references for, 100
  for relieving depression, 257–258
  risks associated with, 136
  safety of, 136
  for slowing blood clot formation, 254–255
  for stopping seizures, 257
  for stress reduction, 173
  therapeutic properties of, 101–103
  for treating anxiety, 259
Traditional Chinese Medicine (TCM), 8–9. *See also* acupressure; acupuncture; cancer treatment; medicinals, TCM; practitioners, TCM; reproduction; treatment, TCM
  anatomy, 35–42
  ancient scrolls, 11–13, 72
  and beliefs, 14
  channels, 42–47
  commitment level of patients, 19
  Eight Balances, 31–35, 103, 122, 195
  Five Elements, 24–31, 35, 48, 195–196, 200, 217, 219
  healing expectations of patients, 18–19
  and holistic medicine, 9–10
  limitations of, 18
  natural healing, 9
  observation of nature, 11, 25
  Qi problems, 47–49
  resources, 277–282
  seeking spiritual guidance, 13
  therapies, 15–17, 95–120
  Vital Three, 21–23, 34–35, 45, 195
  worldwide practice of, 16
transcutaneous electrical nerve stimulation (TENS), 17

WHO. *See* World Health Organization

whole-body approach, 9–10

whole grains, 222

Whole Health system, VHA, 65

Wild Goose Qigong (*Da Yan*), 118

will, 163

Wind (*Feng*), 198–199

Wood, 25–26, 39, 196

World Health Organization (WHO), 63, 84, 141, 188–189

wrong-direction Qi, 49

Wu Wei Zi (Fructus schisandrae chinensis), 259

X

Xiao Mai (Fructus tritici), 257–260

Xie Cao (Radix et rhizome valerianae), 258

xin bao luo. *See* pericardium

Xuan Shen (Radix scrophulariae), 256

Y

Yangbai point, 234

Yang White point, 234

Yee-Kung, Lok, 75

yi, 163

Yin and Yang, 32, 47, 203. *See also* Qi

  equilibrium, 48

  and human anatomy, 36–37, 41

  and TCHs, 102

Yin Qiao (Chiao) San, 241

Yin Qiao Jin. *See* Yin Qiao (Chiao) San

Yintang point, 235–236

Yin-Yang water, 221–222

Yu Jin (Radix curcumae), 255, 259

Yunnan Baiyao, 246

Yu Ping Feng San, 245

Z

Zang organs, 36, 37, 162

Ze Xie (*Rhizoma alismatis*), 256

Zhang Zhenjun, 85

Zheng Gu Shui, 247

zhi, 163

Zhi Mu (Radix anemarrhenae), 256

Zhi Shi (Fructus aurantii immaturus), 254

Zhu Ling (*Polyporus*), 256

Zi Shen Yu Tai Wan, 182–183

zolpidem, 258

About the Author

Mi-Yung Rhee came to the U.S. at age 18 months with permed ringlets because her grandmother thought all American girls looked like Shirley Temple. In third grade, she declared that she wanted to be a writer when she grew up. By the time she graduated from the Medill School of Journalism, she decided she didn't want to be that kind of writer. But writing and proficiency in English as her second language delivered her a 20-plus-year career in marketing. She seems to manifest both her Water Rabbit and Aquarian traits with a preference for calm and stability, yet follows her intellectual curiosity and instinct to upend the norm and take the road less traveled (from her favorite poem, Robert Frost's "The Road Not Taken"). Mi-Yung continues to buck convention by maintaining two careers. She treats patients in her private practice, Healthy Qi & You, as a nationally certified and California-licensed doctor of Traditional Chinese Medicine. Also, she works as a senior marketing manager with MIG, Inc., a national planning and design firm based in Berkeley, California.

Dedication

I dedicate this book to my late parents, Dr. Sang Seol Rhee and Chung-Wha Kim. They survived occupation, colonization, attempts to eradicate their culture, two wars, emigration from Seoul to New York City, prejudice and resentment, and 57 years of marriage. They gave my siblings and me every opportunity to succeed and, in my case, picked me up every time I faltered. This book is as much a result of their love, hard work, and effort as it is mine.

Author's Acknowledgments

There are so many people to acknowledge for this opportunity. I could write another book!

First, my sister Mi-Kyung and brother Joon, who keep their big sister rooted and stable in so many ways.

My family tree of nieces, aunts, uncles, cousins, and so on in the States, South Korea, and other parts of the world, who keep me connected to my culture and heritage.

My found family of lifelong friends, sorority sisters and soul sistahs, godchildren and their parents, schoolmates, roommates, workmates, book mates, and exercise and sports mates whose bonds run true and deep.

Every teacher who taught me the art of expression, the skill of observation, and the love of language from St. Charles Elementary, Eli Terry Elementary, Bridlepath Elementary, Sedgewick Junior High, Shawnee High School, Northwestern University, and the University of California, Berkeley.

The doctors, clinic supervisors, faculty, administrators, and fellow students from the American College of Traditional Chinese Medicine who brought this medicine to life for me and showed me the breadth of its possibilities.

The colleagues who contributed their knowledge and skills to this book: Anna, Arya, Claudia, DaGang, John, and Jung.

My current and former patients who entrust me with their care and continue to allow me to learn.

The Wiley team who presented me with this opportunity and persevered with me through personal loss and health challenges, particularly Jennifer Yee, Donna Wright, Laura Miller, and Colleen Diamond.

Publisher's Acknowledgments

Acquisitions Editor: Jennifer Yee

Managing Editor: Murari Mukundan

Development Editors: Colleen Diamond, Donna Wright

Copy Editors: Laura Miller, Rick Kughen

Technical Editor: Anna Ritner

Production Editor: Magesh Elangovan

Cover Image: © XH4D/Getty Images